Integrating a Palliative Approach:
ESSENTIALS FOR PERSONAL SUPPORT WORKERS

Integrating a Palliative Approach:
ESSENTIALS FOR PERSONAL SUPPORT WORKERS

Katherine Murray

RN, BSN, MA, CHPCN(C)

Life and Death Matters
Victoria, BC

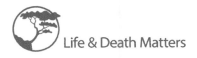

Life & Death Matters

www.lifeanddeathmatters.ca

Published by Life and Death Matters, Victoria, BC, Canada
www.lifeanddeathmatters.ca

Illustrations by Joanne Thomson
Editing by Sarah Weber
Design by Greg Glover

Library and Archives Canada Cataloguing in Publication

Murray, Katherine, 1957-, author
    Integrating a palliative approach : essentials for personal
support workers / by Katherine Murray ; edited by Sarah Weber
; illustrated by Joanne Thomson ; graphic design by Greg Glover.

Includes bibliographical references and index.
Integrating a palliative approach., Workbook.
ISBN 978-1-926923-04-8 (pbk.)

    1. Palliative treatment. 2. Terminal care. 3. Terminally ill--Care.
I. Title.

R726.8.M868 2014   616.02'9   C2014-906911-1

Disclaimer

This book is intended only as a resource of general education on the subject matter. Every effort has been made to ensure the accuracy of the information it contains; however, there is no guarantee that the information will remain current beyond the date of publication. The information and techniques provided in this book should be used in consultation with qualified medical health professionals and should not be considered a replacement, substitute, or alternative for their guidance, assessment, or treatment. The author and publisher accept no responsibility or liability with respect to any person or entity for loss or damage or any other problem caused or alleged to be caused directly or indirectly by information contained in this book.

DEDICATION

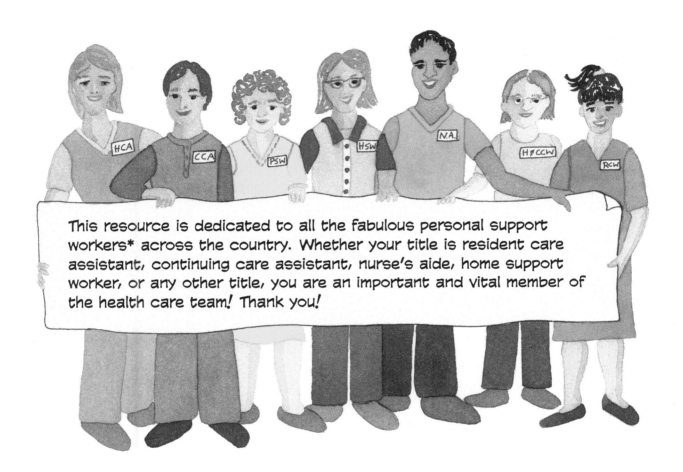

This resource is dedicated to all the fabulous personal support workers* across the country. Whether your title is resident care assistant, continuing care assistant, nurse's aide, home support worker, or any other title, you are an important and vital member of the health care team! Thank you!

*I refer to you as personal support workers throughout this book, but I acknowledge that many of you work under a variety of other titles.

About the Cover

The arbutus tree shown on the cover of this book is native to southeastern Vancouver Island, the nearby Gulf Islands, the adjacent coast of mainland British Columbia, and some areas along the west coast of the United States. Often rooted in the crevices of rock faces along the shore, this tree, with its gnarled and twisted branches, hangs over the edge and is blown about by the wind. The smooth, papery bark peels off as new bark grows. Each arbutus is unique.

The arbutus inspires me with its ability to grow, survive, and even thrive in such rough and rocky areas. This tree graces the cover of my book because to me the arbutus symbolizes the strength of the human spirit, the amazing ability of human beings to survive, grow, and even thrive in difficult, harsh, and even traumatic situations. Like the tree, we too get gnarled as we age. And like the tree, we are all unique.

The arbutus reminds me of those I care for, those who grew in the midst of dying, who grew as they cared for their loved ones or in the years following.

The arbutus reminds me of you, the many personal support workers, health care assistants, continuing care assistants, and so on that I have taught over the years. You also struggle with personal and work challenges, you provide excellent care, and you inspire me with your stories.

I wish you well as you continue on your path of caring for others. I hope that you will find great satisfaction and growth in doing this work.

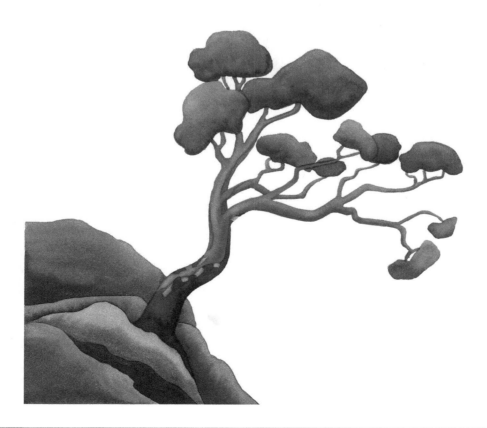

ACKNOWLEDGEMENTS

I joke that my best talent is connecting and pulling together incredible people. And truly, I have been fortunate to work with incredible people throughout the writing of this resource.

Many thanks to Dr. Anne Bruce, Dr. Antoinette Oberg, and the personal support worker (PSW) students and instructors who participated in the evaluation of *Essentials in Hospice Palliative Care: A Resource for Caregivers* and companion study materials in 2013. Your comments informed the changes to this text and my decision to write it specifically for you, PSWs.

Thank you to the hospice palliative care leaders who have assisted with researching, editing, and reviewing the materials. I thank nurses Della Roberts, Terry Downing, Coby Tschanz, Joanne Davidson, and Angela Hope, counsellors Elizabeth Causton, Susan Breiddal, and Misha Butot, physiotherapists Susannah Stewart and Kristina Brown, music caregiver Bev Foster, and physician Joshua Shadd. Thank you to the dementia care nurses Janice Robinson and Fiona Sudbury, and the team at Broadmead Lodge.

I appreciate the expert advice from Lynelle Hamilton, director of the PSW Educational Program Accreditation agency, PSW Jackie McDonald, and PSW educators Karen Mayer, Ann Robinson, Kim Duffus, Katie Cloak, and Leanne McKinzley. Thank you so much. Your understanding of the issues PSWs across Canada face helped me focus on real needs and issues.

Thank you to Elizabeth Causton, Andrea Warnick, Cari Hoffman, and Françoise Mathieu for your contributions. Elizabeth Causton, a hospice palliative care counsellor and educator extraordinaire, contributed to the psychosocial content. Andrea Warnick, a grief counsellor, contributed to the section on supporting children. Cari Hoffman, a national leader in advance care planning, contributed to the section on that subject. Françoise Mathieu, of Compassion Fatigue Solutions and author of *The Compassion Fatigue Workbook: Creative Tools for Transforming Compassion Fatigue and Vicarious Traumatization*, contributed to the chapter on self-care.

I wanted to create a resource that is user friendly and engaging (or as I like to say, "a resource that is delicious and digestible!"). I needed illustrations. How lucky I was to find Joanne Thomson, a gifted West Coast artist, a former nurse, and an adult educator who also taught home support workers for many years! Thank you.

And thank you Greg Glover, graphic designer, for the beautiful book design and layout.

Ann-Marie Gilbert brings her skills as a writer, editor, educator, and computer geek to Life and Death Matters. Ann-Marie's commitment to exceptional resources has pushed me—on more than a few occasions—"back to the drawing board." Thank you, Ann-Marie! Sarah Weber brought "fresh eyes" to this project, which she used to edit this book with precision and care. Thank you!

Ted Murray, my dear and fabulous hubby and partner in Life and Death Matters, is an ongoing source of inspiration and support. Thank you.

Finally and most importantly, I am inspired by you—the PSWs I have met over the years—in the home, in long-term care facilities, in acute care settings, and in workshops and colleges. I am also inspired by those I have not met but have heard about from families and health care professionals. I acknowledge you, I acknowledge the difficult work that you do, and I esteem you. You are amazing! This book is for you. Thank you for sharing yourselves and your stories, and thank you for teaching me.

CONTENTS

PREFACE

I came to hospice nursing as a child. A few of my earliest recollections of death include a dead rat and a lovely transparent leaf. I tried to nurse both back to life, with no success. When my siblings and I found a dead bird, we decided we were not doing well in the healing department and opted for burial.

During my teenage years, I lived with my aunt Frankie. Frankie, a nurse, was the master family caregiver. During my teens she cared for many family members and friends through aging, illness, and dying. I learned that death is a part of life.

As a teen and young adult, I had friends who died. I learned that even the young die. I learned that people die from cancer, accidents, and suicide. (Later I realized that people also die over a longer term, from chronic, progressive, life-limiting illnesses.)

When I was in my 20s, my father and my uncle died. My uncle died after months of excruciating pain, not able to access morphine because, he was told, it needed to be saved for when the pain was "really bad," and because "he might become addicted." My father died with congestion in his lungs, gasping for air. No medications were available to relieve the breathlessness or decrease the congestion.

In the late 1980s, as the hospice palliative care movement spread across North America, I began nursing at Victoria Hospice. I learned about symptoms and symptom management. I learned about loss and grief, last days and hours, rituals, transitions, and traditions. I learned about people, about families, about communication. I became more comfortable talking about dying, grief, loss, and death.

At hospice I had the wonderful blessing of working with a phenomenal team of nurses, physicians, social workers, counsellors, and volunteers. I learned the value of being part of a team. With this team I learned the essentials of hospice palliative care. I learned that much of the suffering that I had witnessed earlier as a friend and as a family member could have been prevented if hospice palliative care principles, practices, and philosophy had been integrated into the care provided.

During these years, I was concerned that only a minority of the dying receive hospice palliative care services. So, it is with delight that I watch as hospice palliative care principles and practices are applied in caring for people with any life-threatening disease. In 2006 I was asked to develop an education program about integrating palliative care into caring for people with dementia. And since that time I have witnessed the international move toward integrating hospice palliative care into caring for people with any life-threatening illness, early in the disease process, across all care settings. The phrase used to describe this is "the palliative approach."

A palliative approach can be integrated into care by all care providers in acute, emergency, long-term, and home care settings. A palliative approach does not need to be provided by specialists. The inclusion of a palliative approach across all settings means that all the dying, not just a minority of them, can benefit from the principles of hospice palliative care.

The purpose of this book is to help you, PSWs, learn and apply the basics of a palliative approach. It is my sincere hope that as you read this book and study using the companion resources, you will feel more confident and competent to provide excellent compassionate care for the dying person[1] and their family.

I wish you well in this learning and invite you to share with me your experiences via the contact link on the Life and Death Matters website (www.lifeanddeathmatters.ca).

Kath Murray
Life and Death Matters
Autumn 2014

---

1 In this text, a person who is dying is referred to as "the dying person" or "the person," and the people the dying person has identified as family, including biological, and chosen family, friends and all significant others, are referred to as "family."

How to Use This Book

When I decided to write this book specifically for you, personal support workers (PSWs), I figured that it would be a small book. Well, surprise, surprise! When I added illustrations and stories, addressed national education standards and provincial learning outcomes, considered the increasing responsibilities that PSWs are assigned, and remembered that you provide the majority of direct care in many settings, the book became much bigger than I had imagined!

Take a deep breath. If you are a PSW student, use the companion workbook as a guide for studying the textbook. The workbook builds on the basics. Do not feel you need to learn everything right now. Follow your instructor's directions about what content you need to know at this point, and what you can put aside to learn in the coming months or years.

If you are a PSW already working in the field, you may want to read this book cover to cover, use it as a reference as you provide care for people and questions arise, or share it with people whose loved ones are dying.

I believe that teaching is an invitation to learn and learning is an invitation to teach. As you learn, share your learning with your colleagues. As you share your learning, you will not only help them learn the importance of integrating a palliative approach into caregiving, but also deepen your own knowledge.

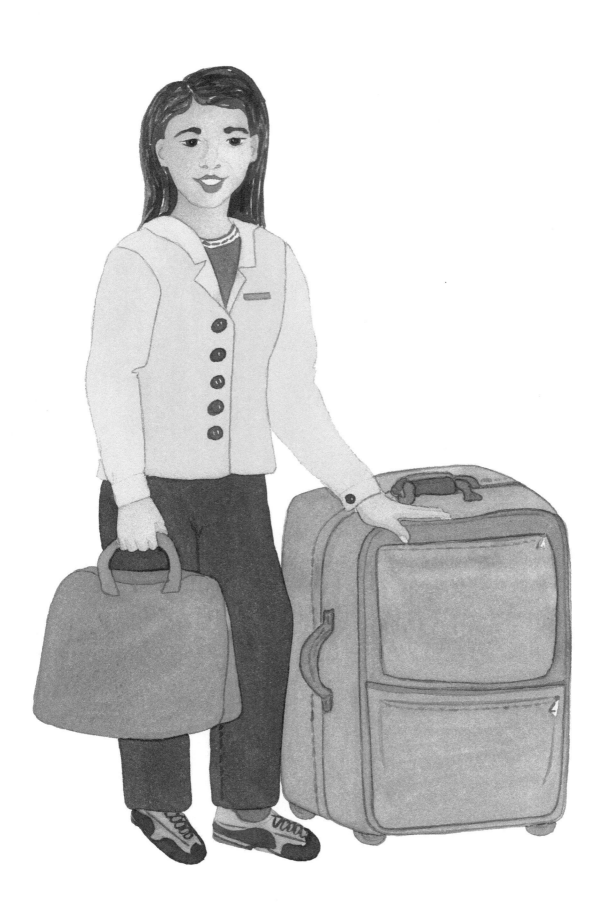

Preparing to Care

Life Is a Journey

Life is often referred to as a journey. I will use the metaphor of the journey throughout this book to refer to the journey of the dying person and their family.[1]

Journey of the dying

As a personal support worker (PSW), you are not the travel guide, the ticket agent, or the pilot for this journey. (Your journey, and the need to attend to your own needs, is discussed in Chapter 7. Self-care, including taking time for reflection, is good for those you care for and good for you.)

I start and end this book with a focus on you, the PSW. Why? Because this book is for you! It is a tool to help you feel more confident and be more competent in providing excellent, compassionate care for the dying and their family. The care you provide for them and your ability to continue to do this work begins and ends with you.

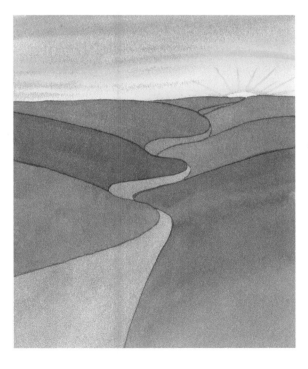

You are invited on a journey. You are invited to journey with people who are dying and their families.

---

1 I use the term "dying person" because I cannot bear to use the word "client" to describe someone who is so vulnerable, I cannot use the word "patient" to describe someone who probably feels anything but patient, and I cannot use the word "resident," as it is not applicable in all care settings.

In this book, "family" means not only people who are related biologically to the dying person, but also chosen family and, for the sake of simplicity, significant others.

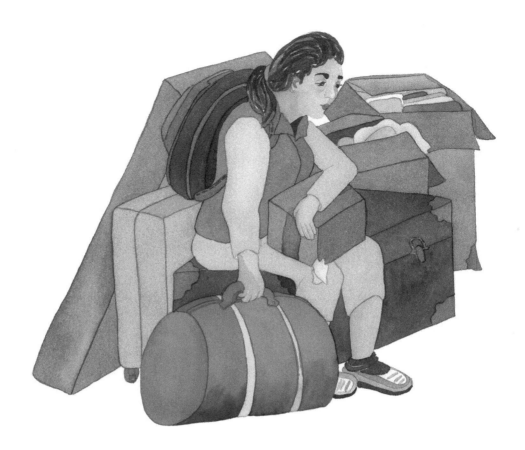

Baggage is values, beliefs, opinions, culture, stereotypes and experiences that you carry with you

You bring baggage with you on this journey. Your values, beliefs, opinions, culture, stereotypes, experiences, and so on make up the baggage that you carry.

Baggage is not good or bad, it is just human to carry it with you.

I encourage you to be aware of what baggage you carry with you and to travel light.

People gather excess baggage.

Excess baggage can get in the way of providing excellent care.

Excess baggage is often those things that people are not aware of.

Regular self-reflection can help you travel light so that you carry only those bags that still have meaning and value to you. Sort your bags and release those things that no longer serve you well.

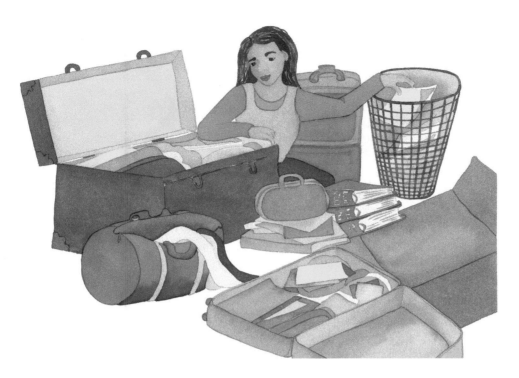

Be aware of those things that you do not want to release but that may negatively affect the care you provide. Awareness will help you avoid tripping over your bags.

Travelling light makes it easier to put your bags to the side and provide excellent care for the dying person and their family.

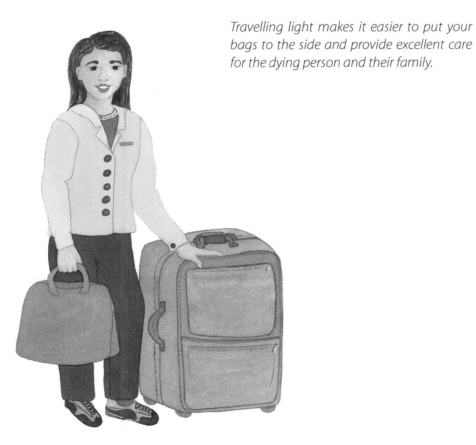

Using Reflection to Develop Self-Awareness

> *Years ago, a wise counsellor (Adaline O'Gorman) taught me this: "You are the greatest gift you bring, but you have to get out of the way so you can do the work!"*

Self-awareness is...

We bring our experiences, values, stereotypes, hopes, dreams, and needs to every encounter in life. For good or bad, they are our baggage, and they direct all our actions and interactions. Self-awareness is the knowledge and acknowledgement of our baggage and its effects on our behaviour and the impact it has on other people.

Why Self-Awareness Is Important

Self-awareness is necessary to provide excellent care. Excellent care is particularly appreciated by the dying person and their family. Why? Because there is no dress rehearsal for the dying; the dying die only once. Memories of witnessing the dying process remain with families for years, perhaps forever. They remember the kindnesses; they also remember insensitive and unkind statements. Meeting the needs of the dying and their family requires self-awareness.

Being aware of your personal baggage and setting it aside

Self-awareness includes being aware of what is in your personal baggage—beliefs, hopes, dreams, experiences, and so on—and then setting it aside in order to provide individualized care that meets the needs of the dying person. You cannot provide effective care for another person's needs if you cannot distinguish between your needs and theirs. Being culturally and spiritually respectful requires that you are aware of your values, stereotypes, and prejudices. Being culturally and spiritually competent requires being able to support people with diverse lifestyles, beliefs, and values. Being aware of your baggage and setting your baggage aside when caregiving allows you to more clearly understand and act on the unique needs and wishes of the person.

> *I was caring for a lady who was dying. One day I bathed her, brushed her teeth, put a clean nightie on her, combed her hair, put clean sheets on her bed, and settled her in her nice clean bed. Then I sat down to read to her. I am not big on the Bible, but she was big on the Bible, so I read to her from her Bible. After I read for a while, I looked up and she wasn't breathing. I didn't know what to do, so I just kept reading from her Bible. I looked up a little while later and she was still dead. I didn't know what to do, so I kept reading from her Bible. I am not big on the Bible, but she was big on the Bible and I read from her Bible and I wondered, "Did I kill her?"*

I remember the PSW who shared this story in a workshop. She told the story with such sincerity and concern. In the end, a bit of humour came forth.

The other students addressed her concern. They applauded her for providing care that respected the individual. They commented on how she put aside her baggage—her lack of interest in the Bible—to provide what was important to the dying woman. Students pointed out to this PSW that she had provided beautiful physical care, and had physically done what the woman needed to be ready to die. The woman was clean and ready to go. They assured the PSW that she had not killed the woman but had provided a safe and secure environment for this woman to die while she was being read to from a book that was so important to her. To use the metaphor of the baggage, the student put aside her baggage to provide personalized care.

The following story illustrates the baggage—the labels and assumptions that a counsellor carried with her about homelessness—and the definition of a "life well lived."

Baggage may be labels and assumptions

> *One day I had the good fortune to meet an elderly woman who had lived on the street for most of her life. While I was quick to judge and pity her for her lack of worldly possessions and stable lifestyle, she spoke of her freedom to be fully present in and open to life, to the experiences and people she met without the distraction of "things." She said that she travelled light in life and that her legacy was in the memories of the generous gifts of time and attention that she left with those she loved. She didn't judge others for their choices and chose not to be defined by those who felt the need to judge her. While I had assumed that this woman had nothing to offer me, her serenity in the face of death taught me a life lesson that I have never forgotten.*

The counsellor reflected on her judgments and assumptions about homeless people. She learned from the woman she was caring for, and moved ahead with new understanding and increased ability to care.

> *He was in his last weeks. He was quiet and withdrawn. I cared for him each day, and I struggled to know how I could connect with this man who did not talk. I knew that he liked to be quiet, so I put a "stopper on my talker." I talked very little as I provided care.*
>
> *When it was quiet on the unit, I would go and sit with him. I would ask, "Do you want me to read, or do you just want me to sit with you?" Often I just sat quietly.*
>
> *One day he said, "I am glad you are here. The nurse yesterday did not stop talking!" I realize that my silence was helpful. When he died, his daughter thanked me and said how he had appreciated the quiet care that I had provided.*

The story above came from a person whose goal is to provide excellent care and to connect with the people she cares for. She told me that by nature she is talkative and energetic. She knew that her normal energy and way of being was not what this gentleman preferred. Because she was aware of her impact on people, and aware of his preferences and needs, she chose to offer a quiet presence. By knowing who you are, you are more able to adapt your behaviour to meet, in the moment, the needs of the person for whom you are caring.

I remember visiting a family at their home, where the only sounds were the dying woman's breathing and a CD playing some very quiet piano music. She took her last breath as the last note of a quiet classical piece sounded and a petal from the last rose of summer fell to the table. At the next home I visited, a man was dying as his daughters played honky-tonk country music on the piano, and the family shared jokes, reminisced, and teased their unresponsive father. In both homes, my presence was required, but I adapted my actions to address the individual needs.

Enhancing Self-Awareness with Reflective Activities

Reflective activities help you sort through your baggage

Self-reflective activities can help you "sort through your baggage." These activities can lead you to explore your inner world, your thoughts, and your feelings, and develop a greater understanding of your motivations—biases, needs, wants, hopes, dreams, and beliefs. (See the companion workbook for reflective activities.)

Maintaining Therapeutic Boundaries

Boundaries are the edges or invisible lines in relationships. Boundaries help you feel deeply but think clearly and act wisely in your work. Boundaries help you care a lot while not "caring too much." When you know the boundaries, you are less likely to get lost in empathy and grief or become cool and distant, cynical and hardened.

Boundaries remind you that you can get very close to the people you care for and still know that their story is not your story. Boundaries help remind you that their life is not your life and their death is not your death.

Boundaries help you to care for the dying

Caring for the dying is difficult. You repeatedly say hello and goodbye. You connect with people, knowing that one day you will disconnect. Maintaining boundaries helps you remember your role, and whose needs you are trying to meet and whose emotions you feel. When boundaries are blurred, it may be more difficult to remember your role, whom you are responsible for, whose needs you are trying to meet, and whose emotions you are feeling.

Maintaining clear boundaries can be particularly difficult for a PSW. The family may expect more from you than is realistic. The dying person and family often struggle to know who is who on the health care team, and may ask you questions or ask you to do things that they should ask the nurse. As you provide the majority of direct care and spend more time with the person and their family than anyone else on the team, they may start to think of you as more like a close friend or family caregiver. They may share with you their concerns, questions, challenges, and fears, ask you for your opinions on treatment issues, and ask you to sign documents. In the home, they may ask you to do housework and prepare meals even if those tasks are not assigned to you in the care plan.

Thinking about boundaries may remind you that while you care deeply about some families, you can acknowledge that you are still an "intimate stranger" in the lives of those you care for. The idea of boundaries may help you remember that the dying person's family is not your family. Although you may feel like family, you are not family; you have not shared the family history, nor have you known this family apart from this experience of illness and loss. You entered their lives in their moment of need, not to become a member of their extended family, but to offer them your expertise in caregiving as part of a job that you have been hired to do.

When you are not clear about boundaries, you may lose your ability to think clearly and act wisely, especially when you are in the presence of strong emotions, difficult family dynamics, or challenging issues related to care of the person who is dying.

<aside>Unclear boundaries may make it difficult to think clearly</aside>

When you care for the dying person and their family, in addition to doing so in moments and situations that are incredible, heart-warming, life affirming, sacred, special, life changing, and so on, at times you will provide care in difficult, painful situations. Boundaries may help you to separate yourself from the suffering, the pain, and the sorrow, and to remember that your job is to support, not to fix. Boundaries may help you remember that, at the end of the day, you will return to the healthy life that you have created.

How Do You Know If Boundaries Are Not Clear?

You experience extreme emotions

Experiencing extreme emotions often indicates that something about the situation or the people in it is resonating with something important, perhaps even unresolved, in your own life. The emphasis here is on an extreme, gut reaction that may even catch you by surprise. This is not the same as the appropriate, shared grief that you may experience in the course of your work.

<aside>3 signs of unclear boundaries in caregiving
1. You feel extreme emotions
2. You feel ownership of patients
3. You try to control</aside>

You feel ownership of patients

Ownership issues arise when you feel unwilling to share "your" patients with other PSWs. For example, you may think,

I am the one who they like the best, and I am the best one to care for them ... no one else can do it as well as I can do it.

A lack of boundaries may be an issue if you find yourself phoning your workplace on your days off to check on a person in whose care you are involved, or feel you are indispensable or you lack trust in your colleagues.

You try to take control

Feeling the need to control a dying person's or their family's decisions about care or treatment is an indication that you may be struggling with boundary issues. Putting pressure on a dying person or their family to behave in a certain way or insisting that they accomplish certain things before death are other signs of blurred boundaries.

> *I cry at everything. I feel like I have no skin. I feel out of control. I feel like I'm giving so much of myself at work I don't have anything left to enjoy or be part of my life at home. My daughter said to me, "Mom, you don't laugh anymore."*

> *I get so angry with people who complain about the smallest things when there are other people who are so gracious even when they are much worse off.*

How Do You Know If Boundaries Are Clear?

When boundaries are clear you may feel...

When boundaries are clear, you may cry with those you care for, but you will know why you are crying. You will share personal information only if it will benefit the person you are caring for. You observe and assess rather than judge and label. You work with your team, communicating to it the strategies that work well for the dying person. You help people know that they will be well cared for even when you are not on duty. You listen to the dying person and their family, do not try to influence their decisions, and let them make decisions that feel right to them.

How Can You Get Better at Maintaining Therapeutic Boundaries?

Paying attention to and valuing personal and work-related boundaries are crucial factors in building healthy relationships and preventing burnout related to the stress of over-involvement. Doing the following will help you become better at maintaining therapeutic boundaries:

Strategies for maintaining your boundaries

- Acknowledge the importance of boundaries.
- Be clear about your scope of practice, job description, and any legal and ethical guidelines relating to the work you do.
- Ask your employer to clarify your job description, responsibilities, tasks, and scope of practice and provide this information to both staff and those you care for. Clear policies and guidelines will decrease the stress of blurred boundaries.
- Reflect on situations that cause strong emotions, talk with a supervisor or colleagues to clarify boundaries, and discuss strategies for maintaining boundaries (see the following text box).
- Engage in self-care because it feels good, and because when you take care of yourself, good boundaries are easier to maintain. Do things you love to do. Find ways to set work aside and enjoy your life. You are worth it (see Chapter 7).

Working from a Therapeutic Distance—the Metaphor of the Family Dance

A family dance is one way to describe the different ways that family members interact with one another.

Imagine a family dance in which the dancers move with one another to the family's own music and rhythm. Consider that this family dance has evolved over generations, as the family created their own history and ways of responding to change and loss.

Now consider the family as its struggles to dance in the face of death. Know that when one participant in the dance either sits down or lies down on the dance floor because of terminal illness, the family modifies its old dance to accommodate the changes. Every step taken on the family dance floor has a reason and a history. Do not assume that the family has no idea what they are doing, much less why they are doing it.

When a family struggles to dance, you may want to get onto the family's dance floor to teach them a new dance, with steps from your family dance. When you do this, you forget that their dance is not your dance. When you step into another family's dance, you lose your unique and valuable perspective and you risk becoming lost in your work. There is great value in staying "on the edge of the dance floor." From the edge of the dance floor you can do the following:

- Observe … from a neutral place, without judgment.
- Explore … Consider what you need to ask and what (more) you need to understand about the dying person or the situation.
- Normalize … Imagine what a healing response would look like and what would help this person and their family feel seen, heard, and validated.
- Preserve the integrity of the family dance.

This is what it means to work from a "therapeutic" or helpful distance.

In addition to the value of being on the edge of the dance floor for the family, being there will help you avoid the stress of over-involvement. Working in this way is healthy for everyone, and that is what makes it therapeutic.

However, experience suggests that it is not easy to stay on the edge of the dance floor. Its border is often fluid, and difficult to identify and define. In addition, everyone has "hooks"—people or situations that touch us in some deep, unconscious place. For example, when you care for someone who is your age, or whose father reminds you of your father, or whose child is the same age as your child, it is easy to be "hooked." Before you even know what's happening, you may find yourself hooked out onto someone else's dance floor, wondering how on earth you got there.

Because people who care for the dying have an obligation to do this work with awareness, it is important that they do their "homework," seeking to identify their own hooks and paying attention to signs that they may have stepped over the line. At the same time, it is important to acknowledge that in all likelihood all caregivers will, at one time or another, become over-involved with a person or family in their care. It is important to know the signs of over-involvement.

Work hard to maintain your boundaries and stay off the dance floor of the dying person. Being aware of your own hooks can help you work from a therapeutic distance.   —*Elizabeth Causton*

The next chapter examines the dying process and the common patterns of how people die.

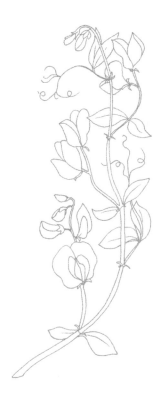

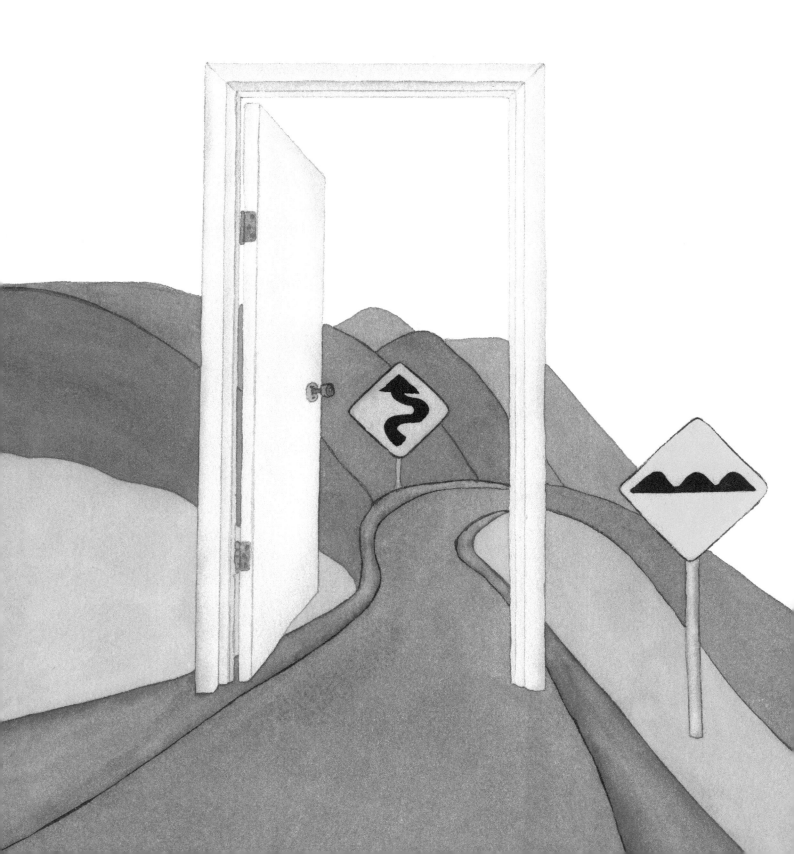

Understanding the Dying Process

People Have Never Died Like This

A hundred or a thousand years ago, people did not die as they die today. In fact, never in known human history have people died as they are dying today.

A hundred years ago, when a farmer got a serious infection, the farmer was either back working in the field or buried in the field a week later. Death was mostly due to infections and occurred over days, sometimes weeks. Dying rarely took months or years.

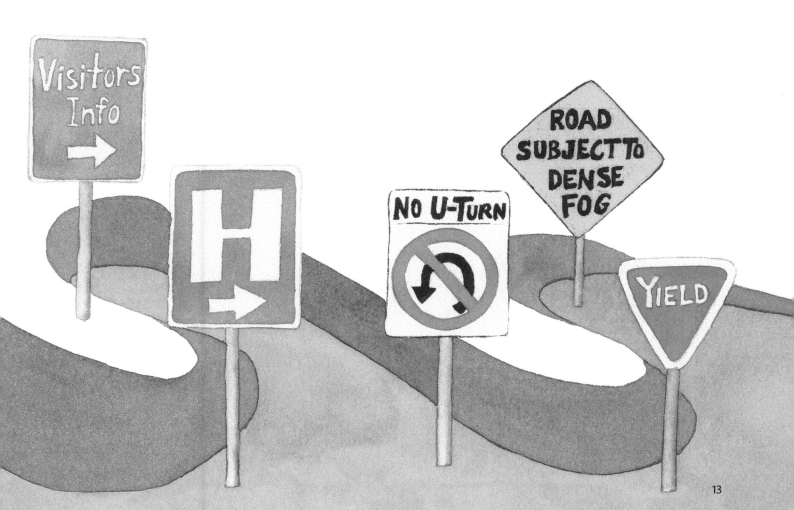

My grandfather was a farmer. One morning he was sick. He worked in the fields all day. At night he was worse. His pain was excruciating. They sent for the doctor. The doctor came in the morning, laid him on the kitchen table, and cut open his abdomen. He was full of gangrene. He died three days later.

Most people die with at least one chronic illness

Advances in medical science have helped people survive illnesses that previously would have killed them. Humans are living longer than ever before, and the process of dying is different than it used to be. Most people die with one or more chronic illnesses require help over a longer time and have fewer caregivers to provide care.

To understand the needs of the dying person and their family, is it important to understand the patterns of dying, to understand that the dying process is more than the physical changes in the last days and hours, and to know that one person's idea of a good death may be another person's idea of a bad death.

Patterns of Dying

Dying is a unique process for each person but usually occurs in one of four patterns: sudden death, steady decline, stuttering decline (the "roller coaster"), and slow decline.

Caregivers observe the functional skills or abilities[1] below to understand the declining condition of a dying person:
- Ambulation (the ability to move around)
- Participation in activities
- Personal care
- Eating and drinking
- Cognitive functioning

Common patterns of dying
• sudden death
• steady decline
• roller coaster
• slow decline

The patterns of decline can be drawn and are known in health care as "trajectories." Each trajectory has different challenges for the dying person and for their family and caregivers.

The stories that follow illustrate the four trajectories and associated challenges. More information on physical comfort care is provided in Chapter 4, psychosocial care in Chapter 5, and care in the last days and hours in Chapter 6.

---

1   A person's level of functioning can be rated on the Victoria Hospice Palliative Performance Scale (PPS) (see page 49). When the level of functioning is observed day after day, week after week, the decline, the rate of decline, and the pattern of decline may become apparent.

Sudden Death

Approximately 10% of people in Canada will die suddenly. Common causes of sudden death include heart attack, major stroke, or car accident. In cases of sudden death (Figure 1), neither the dying person nor their family members know that death is imminent.

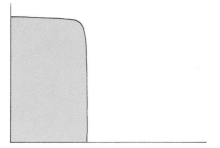

Sudden death trajectory

Figure 1. The sudden death trajectory

Sudden Death

I was playing baseball when my brother called to tell me that our mom had died from a heart attack. I went straight to the hospital but was too late. It is hard to believe. I wish we had been prepared. It would have been easier if she had been sick for a while so that I could have said goodbye and told her that I loved her. I feel like I was hit by a truck!

When I ask people how they want to die, there are always people who say they would prefer a sudden death. They often state that they do not want to be a burden on their loved ones. However, those who have experienced the sudden death of a loved one may grieve the fact that they did not have time to say goodbye or to prepare for or anticipate the death, and may say that they wish they could have provided care. These people may say,

10% of people die of sudden death e.g. heart attack, major stroke or accident

> *Well it might have been a good death for her, but it was not a good death for me.*

As a PSW you may witness a sudden death or arrive just after a sudden death. Chapter 6 provides information on what to do after a sudden unexpected death has occurred.

Steady Decline

The steady decline pattern of dying (Figure 2) often occurs in people dying from cancer. These individuals are relatively strong for a long period, even for years after their diagnosis. They may have a slight decline in functioning when illness recurs and during treatment, and then they experience a significant steady decline in function and strength in the last six months of life. They may be confined to bed only in the last weeks before death.

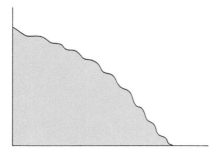

Figure 2. The steady decline trajectory

The story of Yetta's[2] dying illustrates this steady decline. Because her death was anticipated, there was opportunity for Yetta (my mother) and our family to prepare, share, and care. Yetta was grateful to know that she was dying. We talked about what we called the "death benefits." The family gathered. She chose what she wanted to do with her limited energy and time. She registered with the provincial hospice program. People brought food and offered assistance. Cards and emails arrived with expressions of gratitude and stories of a life well lived. As a family, we cared for her and prepared for her dying. My sister sewed a blanket to wrap her body in following death, while my brothers and husband built a beautiful coffin. We coordinated care for a few months. There were only a few sleepless nights.

As much as the steady decline felt like a benefit to Yetta and our family, there are times when the decline can feel too fast and people do not feel they have time to prepare. They may feel that every week they become accustomed to the new normal only to have the person decline again. The decline may feel too fast if the health care team does not explain to the person and the family that the person is dying, or if they explain but the person or family is not ready or able to process the information. The decline may also feel too fast if there are great differences in how individual family members hear and act on the information received.

Most people believe that a steady decline is how most people die. In fact, less than 20% of people die in this way.

---

2 Yetta was insistent that if anything she experienced in dying could help even one person, we, her family, were to share it. I will share a few of her stories throughout this text and know how pleased she would be if you find value in them.

Steady Decline

On the 12th of September Yetta walked 12 kilometres—not bad for an 82-year-old. But 10 weeks later she felt unwell and visited the doctor.

"Fatigue," she said. "Oh, and my right side is sore."

"And you are jaundiced—the whites of your eyes are a bit yellow," the doctor said.

On the 8th of November she was told that the ultrasound showed a tumour, and the next morning a stent was inserted to help the bile flow from her gall bladder. By the afternoon, after a CT scan, the surgeon sat at the end of her bed and very gently and kindly told her, "You have an inoperable tumour."

"How long?" she asked.

"Mm … maybe 6 to 12 months … I hope you will have a good winter."

She was glad that she was not offered any surgery to remove the tumour. She said, "I have to die anyway, so whether I die in six months or in nine months does not really matter."

She got busy, as busy as her energy would allow her. She organized papers and cleaned her desk. She wrote a letter about democratic process to a community group, and resigned as the treasurer. She asked her sister to complete a sweater that she was knitting. She connected with a few old friends she was concerned about. And she connected with her closest friends.

Within six weeks we, her four kids, gathered from around the globe and celebrated Christmas. She talked about the light in a season of darkness. She ate whipping cream. She decided life was too short for cheap wine and decided to eat and drink only what she loved, nibbling small bits of anything she felt like eating and nothing else.

"What do you want? What is important to you in dying? How can we help you?" I asked. She was very clear, "I do not want any pain."

Another few weeks passed. She slept more and got up less. She became unstable on her feet. She said, "I know my date. Next week. Between the 14th and 17th of January." She came close to death a number of times, but then she perked up and started breathing regularly again.

Repeatedly she described her last months as "the richest period of my life."

And then, on the 16th of January in the quiet of the night, she took her last breaths and was gone.

Stuttering Decline—the Roller Coaster

The stuttering trajectory (Figure 3) describes people who alternate between periods of decline and periods of recovery. The period of decline may result from a worsening of chronic illness or be caused by a fall, a fracture, the flu, and so on. At times, the person may require hospitalization and treatment, or they may simply require an adjustment of medications to help them stabilize. Following treatment and stabilization, the person recovers some of their previous level of functioning and may again enjoy activities they used to do. The person may be stable for weeks or months, and then decline again when their chronic illness changes or they experience another infection, fall, or flu. Eventually, the repeated declines lead to death. Approximately 70% of people follow a stuttering decline or a slow decline to death.

~ 70% of people die after a stuttering decline

Stuttering decline trajectory

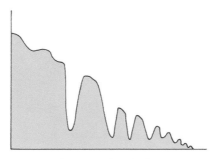

Figure 3. The stuttering decline trajectory

Characterizes dying with organ failure e.g. lung, heart, liver or kidney disease

People with organ failure such as congestive heart failure (CHF), chronic obstructive pulmonary disease (COPD), or end-stage kidney disease, as well as people with chronic progressive illnesses such as Parkinson's disease or dementia-related illnesses, are likely to experience this type of stuttering decline.

Sarah's story illustrates the roller coaster experiences of caring for Tom over the past decade. Sarah talks of her fatigue and the challenge of not knowing the future. When Tom improves, she wonders if he is getting better. Each time he declines, she wonders if he is dying.

It is usually very difficult to estimate the time remaining until death for people in stuttering decline. It is estimated that half of the people with advanced progressive illnesses will not know the week before they die that this will be their last week. Even the day before they die, many individuals will be thought to have up to six months to live.

Michelle Dale, a hospice counsellor, reflecting on her own caregiving experiences, writes,

> *How do you prepare when you don't know if you are running a 100-metre race or a marathon? And how do you train when you don't even know that you were about to run a race at all?*

Stuttering Decline—the Roller Coaster

My name is Sarah. I am Tom's wife and caregiver. Tom has chronic obstructive pulmonary disease, and although we have been dealing with it for over 15 years, the last eight years have been the hardest, with repeat hospital admissions, decreased abilities, and increased needs. I have heard it said that the typical patient with this disease goes to death's door a number of times before dying. At least five times the children have gathered to say goodbye.

June 9: Last week the doctor came in and, squatting to make eye contact with Tom, asked us what we wanted. Tom said that he was tired—tired of hospitals, emergencies, tests, and more treatments. I very carefully suggested hospice. Tom and the doctor agreed.

June 15: We came home by transport ambulance. All the kids came home to help. In the middle of the night, I wept. I am exhausted. I wonder if he will die soon. I hope he will. I hope he won't.

July 15: How long will this go on? It has already been eight years! The personal support workers come five times a week now. I willingly let them help. Tom seems to enjoy them.

July 18: My, oh my, what a journey! This man of mine has always had a huge appetite. Now he is eating so little. It is hard for him to eat and digest and breathe at the same time. I try to feed him but even with all my effort, he eats very little.

August 9: Tom has been restless for the last three nights. He sits on the edge of the bed, tries to get up, then sits down. Then he wants up. We need to be with him because he is unsafe. He has more difficulty breathing. He is confused, sometimes talking to people who aren't there. The other day he dreamt of his mom who died several years ago. His sentences are not making sense, his words jumbled. He was like this last year when he was really sick. He recovered then. I don't think he will recover this time.

August 17: We celebrated our 60th anniversary two months early.

August 19: Tom is very weak, can manage sips of water. He is confused again.

August 20: It is with a sad heart that I tell you my Tom died this morning. He has been sick for 15 years.

Slow Decline

The slow decline trajectory (Figure 4) happens over years. Although there may be periods of decline and improvement, like those seen in the stuttering decline trajectory, the ups and downs in a slow decline are more subtle. The highs are not as high and the lows are not as low, making the decline seem gradual. However, the people who are providing direct care or are involved daily with the dying person may notice the small changes. When the person has a good day, the family may wonder whether they are getting better, and when the person has a bad day, whether death is near.

Slow decline trajectory

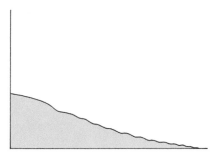

Figure 4. The slow decline trajectory

Parkinson's disease, dementia-related illnesses, and frailties cause this type of slow decline in a person's abilities. With the slow trajectory, people often lose the ability to care for themselves long before they are imminently dying. Unless they develop a significant infection or other medical crisis, people may linger for years. In these cases, the time until death is very difficult to estimate.

Usually, dying people who suffer from Alzheimer's disease first lose their ability to do tasks that require higher levels of thinking, such as balancing a chequebook. Then they gradually lose basic-level functioning, such as being able to do their own personal care, or walk or eat independently. If the person lives long enough, they will lose the most basic abilities, including the ability to swallow.

Characterizes dying with chronic disease e.g. dementia, Parkinson's

People with other types of dementia may experience a differently shaped decline. People with vascular dementia may experience a small stroke that results in a decline in functioning (a step down) and then stabilize (a plateau) until the next stroke occurs. Death may occur following a stroke.

Dying with dementia has been called "death by a thousand deaths." This speaks of the many, many losses experienced by the individual, the family, and the caregivers.

Caregivers struggle to carry the caregiving load over years and may experience fatigue and depression. Consequently, most people with dementia die in long-term care facilities.

Slow Decline

Mom was diagnosed with Parkinson's disease nine years ago, and with Alzheimer's disease five years ago. She did pretty well for the first years, with only a few visits to the doctor. But over the years it got more difficult to care for her. First, she would leave the house and go walking. Then she would get lost, so I had to go with her. Then she would just wander and not really go anywhere, but there was the possibility that she would get lost. Then she did not want to go anywhere or do anything. She started to resist care. She got restless and sometimes agitated and stopped finding pleasure in the cat, stopped watching TV, and did not like to be read to anymore.

At some point, the nurses assessed her and followed up with sending personal support workers to help her with bathing and meals. Volunteers from the local dementia care program provided some respite care. I appreciated this help, but it was not enough. Nights were long; I slept poorly and got up too frequently. Then she fell, cut herself, and bruised her hip. She went by ambulance to emergency and then into a care home.

It was absolutely the most difficult thing I have ever done, leaving her there. I came home and wept. I was so tired of caregiving, but it was still hard to give the caregiving to someone else. And the staff, well, they seem fine, but there are so many of them.

Now, she does not know me. It is as if she is dead—but her body is still here. When I sing to her she becomes agitated. She does not participate in any activities.

She has bladder infections regularly. She hardly eats anything. She has difficulty swallowing. And sometimes does not eat at all. Last month they thought she was dying, but they have thought that before … I sometimes wonder if she will outlive me.

When I think of the positives of the slower decline, I am reminded of Colleen and Del McCarthy, who have been caring for their husband/father who has Parkinson's disease for over 25 years. Recently, he fell and fractured a hip, and then a few months later fell and broke the other hip. Currently he requires total care, medications every two and a half hours during the day, tube feeds three times a day, and regular transfers to the commode. Through it all he has retained his incredible sense of humour. Colleen remarked to me, "I would not trade this time of caregiving for anything. The time with Dad has been so precious." They are assisted by the contribution of fabulous PSWs who provide care five days a week.

Ambiguous dying syndrome

Mercedes Bern-Klug coined the term "ambiguous dying syndrome" to describe those things that happen when a person is dying but the expected time of death is not certain.[3] The ambiguity means that people do not get the "death benefits"—the "benefits of dying"—that people get when death is expected. The ambiguity means that these people are not registered with the palliative benefits programs and do not receive the services of hospice volunteers. They may miss opportunities for life review and closure. They may not have the conversations about what they want when death nears. And by the time death is certain, in the last days and hours, they may be unable to have these conversations.

When the person recovers from near-death repeatedly, the person, family, and health care team may forget that dying is eventually going to occur. When this happens, death may come as a surprise. It is then that the obituary in the newspaper reads, "died suddenly at 94 with COPD, CHF, and dementia."

---

3 M. Bern-Klug, "The Ambiguous Dying Syndrome," *Health and Social Work* 29, no. 1 (2004): 55–65.

The Dying Process

To be able to provide the best support possible to the dying person and their family, PSWs need to understand both the patterns of dying and the physical changes that occur in the last days and hours (see Chapter 6).

Caring for the Dying—Like Running a Race

I've often said to families that caring for the dying is like running a race in which the distance keeps changing. For example, at the time of diagnosis my aunt and my family were all shocked, convinced (due to the words of the doctor) that she had a very short prognosis. We were in a 100-metre sprint.

Everyone came, everyone called and sent letters and flowers, and made declarations of love.

Nobody was thinking about pacing.

And then things changed. It became clear that we were in, maybe, a 10-kilometre race. She had a treatment plan. There was hope being offered by her oncologist. We needed to slow down. We wished we had trained.

Then she had the surgery and it was awfully hard and everyone moved in again. We were back in a short-distance mentality—maybe not a 100-metre dash, maybe an 800-metre race. We needed to give everything, but we had to save a little for the finish.

Now she is doing well again. The prognosis is uncertain. There is talk of survival. Everyone realizes that we are in a marathon. Nobody trained. Someone needs to take responsibility for the water and food station. We need volunteers to stand at the tricky corners to make sure we don't get lost.

As hospice workers we are the ones at the tricky corners.

We don't need to run the race, but we need to know how hard it is. We need to know how confusing and exhausting it is when the finish line keeps getting moved. Imagine being in a marathon and having 2 miles to go and then seeing a new sign that says, "Only 10 miles to go." How does one continue?

— Michelle Dale

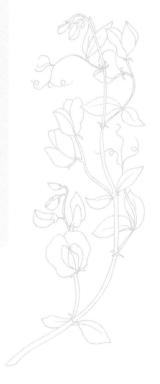

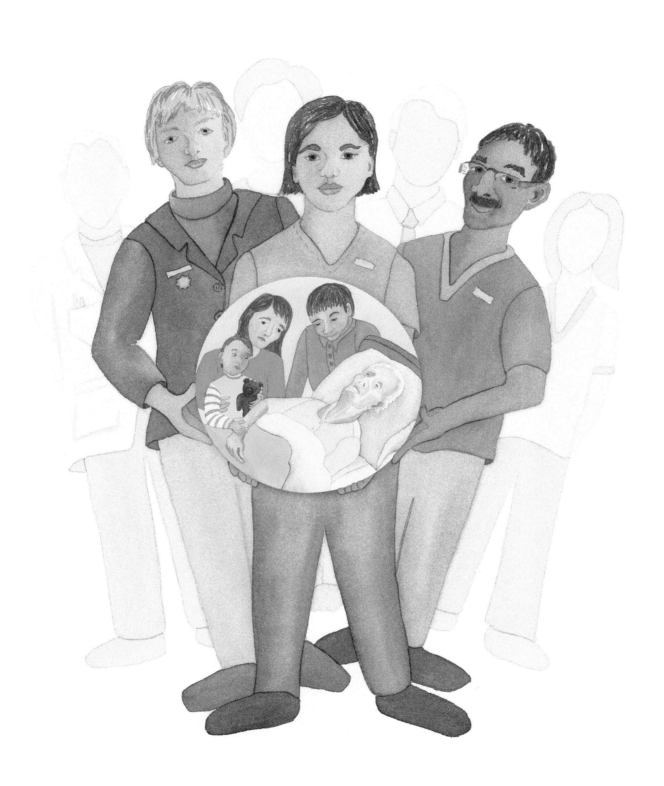

![3]

Integrating a Palliative Approach into Caregiving

The Beginning of Better Care for the Dying

It was the 1960s, and David Tasma was dying in an acute care hospital in London, England. The focus of acute care was not on providing individualized care for the dying person. David talked for hours with his social worker, Cicely Saunders (a former nurse, honoured by Queen Elizabeth II in 1979 with the title Dame Commander of the Order of the British Empire), about a better way to care for the dying. After he died, Cicely completed a medical degree. She built on those early discussions with David to establish a new way of caring for the dying. In 1967, Cicely Saunders opened St. Christopher's Hospice, a facility providing care specifically for dying people, and simultaneously started the hospice movement. This movement has expanded to address the needs of the dying throughout the world.

Cicely Saunders founded St Christopher's Hospice in London, England

Hospice Palliative Care

Dr. Balfour Mount, a Quebec physician, studied in England with Cicely Saunders so that he could better understand the needs of people in his hospital who were dying. He created the term "palliative care" because the word "hospice" did not translate well into French. He opened the palliative care unit in 1974 at the Royal Victoria Hospital in Montreal. In Canada, the terms "hospice" and "palliative" are often used together.

Dr Balfour Mount created the term "Palliative Care"

One goal of hospice palliative care (HPC) is to improve a person's quality of life. Two recent studies support the role of HPC in reaching this goal. A study reported by the Canadian Hospice Palliative Care Association (CHPCA) states that people receiving HPC reported better quality of life, fewer symptoms, and greater satisfaction with care. They also had fewer emergency room visits and fewer hospitalizations.[1] Another study indicated that people receiving palliative care in addition to oncological treatments reported better quality of life.[2] Although HPC is not aimed at helping

Hospice palliative care seeks to improve a person's quality of life

---

1 Paraphrased from Canadian Hospice Palliative Care Association, *A Model to Guide Hospice Palliative Care: Based on National Principles and Norms of Practice*, revised and condensed ed. (CHPCA, 2013), 6.

2 J.S. Temel et al., "Early Palliative Care for Patients with Metastatic Non-Small-Cell Lung Cancer," *New England Journal of Medicine* 363, no. 8 (2010): 733–742.

people live longer, this study found that people who also received palliative care also lived a few months longer than those who did not receive HPC.

> HPC helps people manage symptoms caused by any life-threatening disease.
>
> Life-threatening diseases include end-stage kidney, cardiac, respiratory, and neurological illnesses, as well as dementias, and congenital and metabolic illnesses that occur mostly in children.
>
> People benefit from HPC early in their disease process, sometimes as early as the time of diagnosis. Early in the disease, HPC can help a person by providing information about the disease process, advance care planning, current care options, and support for psychosocial issues.
>
> A person can receive palliative care while still receiving acute curative treatments.
>
> These two approaches, curative and palliative, can work together to provide better quality of life for people with life-threatening diseases.

In hospice palliative care, curative and palliative approaches can work together

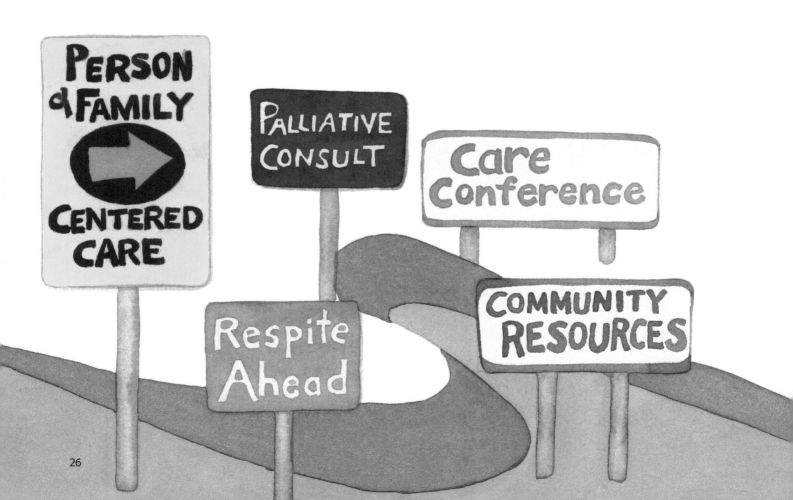

Principles of Hospice Palliative Care

HPC is care that

- Affirms life
- Regards dying as a normal process
- Considers the dying person and their family to be the unit of care and continues through death and bereavement

HPC principles promote care that

- Does not speed or delay dying or death
- Improves the dying person's quality of life
- Provides pain relief and manages distressing symptoms
- Attends to the person's needs in a holistic way

HPC is best when provided by an interprofessional team. The diverse perspectives and abilities of the members of the team enable it to provide holistic care.

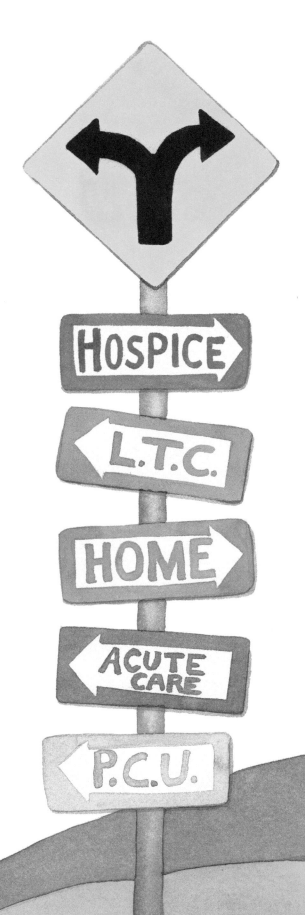

Hospice Is about Living Well Until Death

Around the world, HPC is based on the common philosophy of improving the quality of life for dying people, wherever they are—at home, in a care facility or hospital, or in a palliative care unit. People often say, "Hospice is all about living and living well until you die."

HPC is holistic care that addresses the needs of the entire person—the physical, emotional, spiritual, and psychosocial needs. HPC includes care for whomever the person who is dying defines as "family." The illustration at the beginning of this chapter depicts person- and family-centred care: the caregivers and the health care team are holding the person and family gently, supporting them with compassion and respect for their unique personal experience. Ideally, an interprofessional team that includes PSWs, volunteers, nurses, physicians, social workers, and spiritual care personnel provides HPC.

HPC acknowledges that dying is a normal process and that people often need support to cope with feelings of loss and grief. HPC may include medical tests and interventions to provide comfort, and therefore is appropriate early in an advancing chronic or terminal disease process. People do not need to wait until death is imminent to benefit from HPC.

A Palliative Approach

In Canada, less than 30% of people who are dying receive HPC from HPC specialists. Even fewer people receive grief and bereavement services.[3] Among the reasons why many dying people do not receive specialty HPC services are that there are few specialty teams that provide these services, and most providers of specialty services are located in urban areas.

If you consider the patterns of dying discussed in Chapter 2, you might also predict that people who do access specialty HPC services are those whose pattern of dying is a steady decline and whose time until death is somewhat predictable. People who are less likely to receive such services are those whose pattern of decline is either stuttering or slow and whose time until death is less predictable.

Australia defines "a palliative approach"

In response to these challenges, Palliative Care Australia recommends that a "palliative approach" be integrated in ongoing care provided by the generalist primary care team. The generalist team includes the local primary care physician and direct care nurses. Palliative Care Australia suggests that the generalist team can provide good care to over 65% of dying people.[4]

Current research in Canada[5, 6] suggests that quality palliative care can be provided as part of long-term care by integrating a palliative approach from the time a person moves into long-term care. The principles of a palliative approach dovetail seamlessly with excellence in dementia care. This is especially helpful because people are moving into long-term care residences later in the disease process, often suffering from multiple illnesses. The average length of stay in long-term care is decreasing, and more deaths occur in long-term care settings each year. In many provinces the average length of stay is less than 18 months. Integrating a palliative approach can help ensure that these residents benefit from HPC.

Benefits of integrating a palliative approach

Likewise, many people repeatedly enter the emergency department and acute care in their last six months of life. A focus on integrating a palliative approach can help remind the health care team to share information that will help the person and their family make informed decisions, consider goals of care, make plans to address further decline in health, and be better prepared for the dying process.

A palliative approach, for our purpose

For the purposes of this book, a palliative approach is an approach that integrates the principles, practices, and philosophy of HPC into the care of people with any life-threatening disease, early in the disease process, across all care settings.

---

3 CHPCA, *CHPCA Fact Sheet—Hospice Palliative Care in Canada,* updated March 2014, http://www.chpca.net/media/330558/Fact_Sheet_HPC_in_Canada%20Spring%202014%20Final.pdf.

4 Palliative Care Australia, http://palliativecare.org.au.

5 Initiative for a Palliative Approach in Nursing (iPANEL). Evidence and Leadership (Victoria, BC: University of Victoria), http://www.ipanel.ca/.

6 Palliative Alliance (Quality Palliative Care in Long Term Care), http://www.palliativealliance.ca/.

End of Life Care

Over the past few decades, a new phrase—"end of life"—has increasingly been used to refer to the period of time before death. Some people may find this a more gentle way of talking about the time when death is nearing. However, the phrase does not have a standard definition. Some people use the phrase to refer to the last year or so of life, while others use it to refer to the last weeks of life. If you use this phrase, you may want to clarify what you mean, and if others use the phrase, you may want to ask them what they mean by it. How the phrase is defined will determine what "end of life care" means.

In this book I will use the term "end of life" to refer to the last weeks and days of life.

End of life refers to the last weeks and days of life

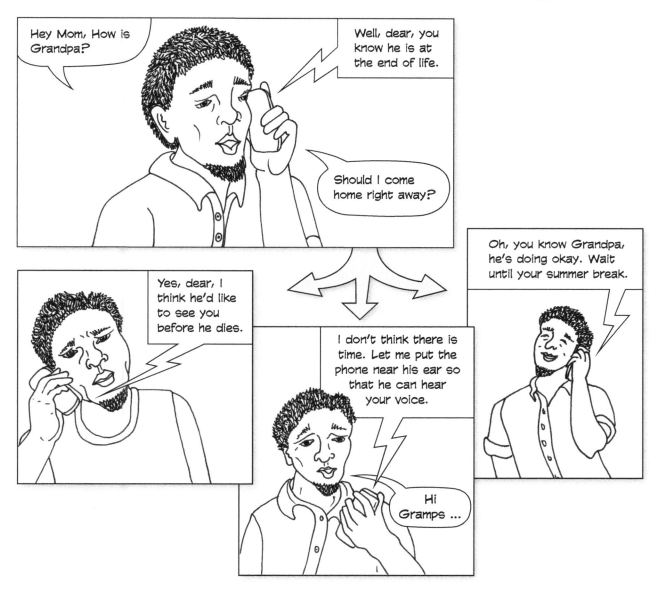

Terms Used in Hospice Palliative Care

Hospice palliative care terms defined for this book

The principles of HPC identify the focus of care and how care is best provided. However, programs across Canada vary in how they use the terms "hospice," "palliative," and "hospice palliative care." In this book, the meanings of these and related terms are as defined below.

End of life care: Care provided in the last weeks and days of life.

Hospice: A program of care provided to people whose death is expected in less than six months, or to the bereaved. The term is also used to refer to the place in which the care is provided.

Hospice society: An organization that offers services such as counselling and volunteer support for the dying and bereaved.

Palliative care: Care that is available to people early in their disease process. It is likely to be provided at the same time as acute curative treatments.

Palliative care units: Areas in acute care hospitals where support for symptom management is provided. When both palliative care and hospice care are available, a person could move from a palliative care unit into a hospice residence as their disease progresses and death nears.

Palliative care beds: Beds in a long-term care facility, set apart from others, to provide care for people who are expected to die in the coming months or weeks.

Palliative consult team: A team of specialists who consult with people about palliative care.

Provincial hospice benefit programs: Government programs that pay for certain medications and equipment for people who are dying at home.

Residential hospice: An inpatient unit or home where dying people can live their last months or weeks.

Palliative approach: An approach that integrates the principles, practices, and philosophy of HPC into the care of people with any life-threatening disease, early in the disease process, across all settings.

Because people vary in how they use these terms, you might ask people to clarify what such terms mean to them.

According to the World Health Organization, "Palliative care is an approach that improves the quality of life of patients and their families facing the problems associated with life-threatening illness, through the prevention and relief of suffering by means of early identification and impeccable assessment and treatment of pain and other problems, physical, psychosocial and spiritual."[7]

Palliative care as defined by the WHO

> **"Palliative" Describes a Type of Care**
>
> Sometimes people label a person in their last days as "palliative": "He's palliative." "She's palliative."
>
> Consider using these phrases instead: "We would not be surprised if he died soon." "He is in his last days and hours."
>
> Use the term "palliative" only when referring to a type of care, a philosophy of care, an approach to care. Do not use it to label a person.
>
> Consider using the terms used in the Victoria Hospice Palliative Performance Scale to describe the person: "He is 10%."

People are not palliative. Care is palliative.
—*Chris Sherwood*

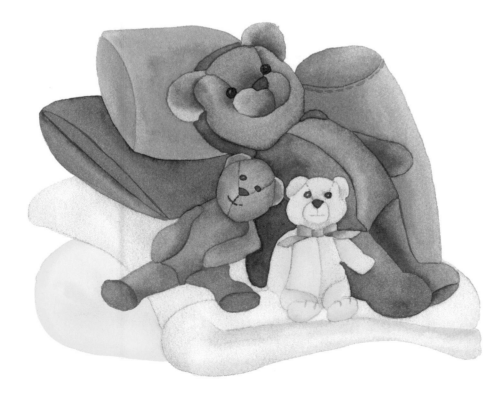

---

7   WHO Definition of Palliative Care, http://www.who.int/cancer/palliative/definition/en/

The Health Care Team

I asked Joanne Thomson to create illustrations for this book with the hope that they would help visual learners understand the concepts it discusses. Since childhood I have been told that "a picture says a thousand words," and so it is with Joanne's paintings. I am thrilled with the illustration for this chapter showing the concept of "team." Joanne and I talked about the person and family being the focus of care, and the work that family caregivers do in providing care for their loved ones, and we spoke about the invaluable contributions PSWs make. The afternoon we talked, I think I held my arms out and suggested that the PSW "holds" the family in a safe, warm embrace, an embrace that is not tight, that allows space for the person and the family to do their work, but that also creates a safe place. We talked of the fact that PSWs often provide care in isolation in the home setting, or with backup support in long-term care facilities. We talked of the team that is available but is often in the background, responding only when called on. This is the illustration that evolved from our discussion. Thank you, Joanne!

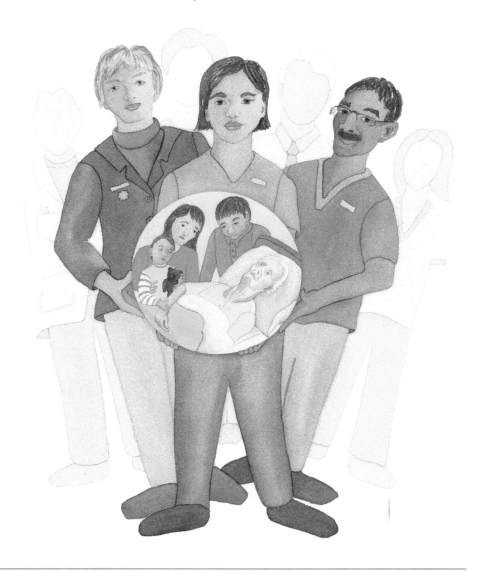

These are the key messages I take from this illustration:

- The dying person and their family are the unit of care.
- The PSW (or other member of the team) "holds" and supports the person and family.
- The image of "holding" suggests care and the creation of a safe, comfortable place.
- The PSW (or other member of the team) is supported by colleagues—in this illustration, another PSW and a nurse who is available to answer questions and address concerns and changing needs.
- The larger team is less visible and may be spread out geographically, but it is available for care or consultation.
- The team will need to communicate well in order to collaborate and provide coordinated and consistent care across the distance.
- The PSW will need to communicate changes in the dying person and their needs, fears, concerns, and questions to the health care team so that care plans can be adapted as needed.

Dying person and their family are the unit of care

You may see other messages in this illustration. I welcome your thoughts.

The health care team is partly determined by where the dying person lives, the services available, and the people who provide those services. The team is also determined by the preferences of the dying person and their family. They may appreciate a big team of people assisting them to meet their goals, or they may want only a few people directly involved in their care.

Health care team is determined by the patient, their location and care needs.

> *When she was pregnant, she learned she had a terminal illness. She enjoyed the short weeks that she had with her newborn baby. As death drew near, the community responded—friends, neighbours, the hospice, the physician, the home care nurse, all were willing to provide support. She chose to limit her team to her close family, a few friends, the physician, and two home care nurses. She did not want anyone else involved. She died supported by her team, with her family around her.*

In a larger urban centre, the interprofessional team may include these and other people: primary care nurses, a hospice nurse and counsellor, a family physician and a hospice physician for consultation, disease-specific specialists, agencies, pharmacists, volunteers, physiotherapists and occupational therapists, music and recreation therapists, activity workers, a dietitian, a kitchen team, friends, extended family, spiritual leaders, a naturopath, a chiropractor, and so on.

When the team is large, the dying person and their family can become very confused as to who is who. They may find it exhausting to answer the same questions asked by different people and may ask, "Don't you people talk with each other?" They may be very stressed if they receive conflicting information from different members of the team.

PSWs provide the
majority of direct care
for the dying in long
term care and possibly
in other care settings

As a PSW, you are an important and valuable member of the health care team. You provide most of the direct care in long term-care settings and much of the direct care in the home (depending on the support family members offer). More and more you are providing care in acute care hospitals. In the early stages of a dying person's decline, you may provide care a few times a week for the person and their family; by the time death is imminent, a team of PSWs may be in the home or at the bedside full-time. You provide care under the direction of a health care professional, usually a nurse, and you work as a member of the larger health care team. As such, you must be skilled not only in providing care, but also in communicating with and participating in the larger team.

You provide support and integrate a palliative approach when you do the following:

What PSWs can do to
integrate a palliative
approach

- Hold the dying person and family at the centre of care
- Consider the needs of the whole person
- Observe, listen, ask, reflect, and respond
- Implement the care plan
- Personalize comfort measures
- Provide physical and psychosocial support
- Communicate and advocate

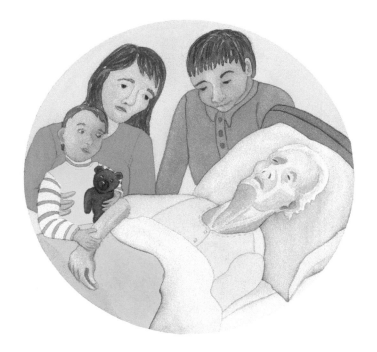

What Is a Good, Bad, or Appropriate Death?

As you look at ways to integrate a palliative approach into caregiving, it is import-ant to know what the dying person wants, and how that person defines "a good death" or "a bad death." The lists in the illustration below show PSWs' responses to the question, "What would be a bad death/good death for you?"

Good death,
Bad death,
Appropriate death

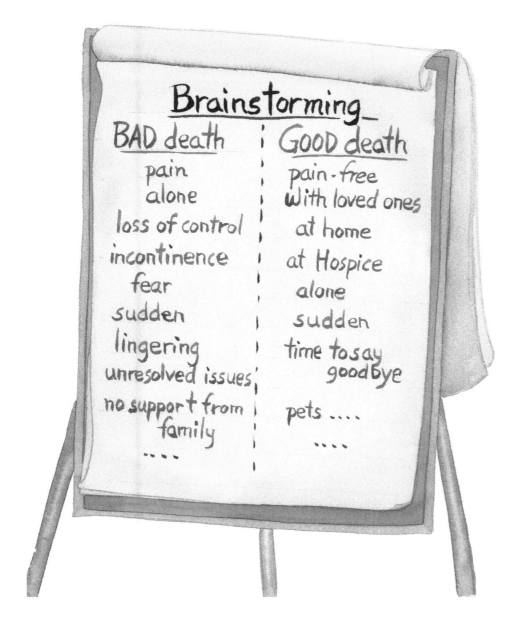

Brainstorming

BAD death	GOOD death
pain	pain-free
alone	with loved ones
loss of control	at home
incontinence	at Hospice
fear	alone
sudden	sudden
lingering	time to say
unresolved issues	goodbye
no support from family	pets ....
.. .. ..	....

It is interesting to note that some items are on only one list while other items are on both lists, which indicates that what makes a good death for one person might be a bad death for someone else.

Rather than use the words "good" or "bad" to describe a death, you may want to think about the phrase "an appropriate death." An appropriate death is one with dignity, where the needs of the dying person are addressed by the team. The term "appropriate death" is not intended to be a judgment. In the following story, a daughter talks about how badly she felt about her mother's death, until she learned the concept of an appropriate death.

For years, I felt badly that Mom had died before I got back to the hospital. The staff had phoned me to tell me that Mom was declining, and I asked them to tell her that I was on my way. She died just before I got there. For years, I felt guilty that I was not with her when she died.

When I heard about an "appropriate death," I remembered that she was a very private person and had always protected us from seeing or experiencing difficult things. When I remembered that, I thought, "Wasn't that just like her to die when I wasn't there!" With this new understanding, I felt at peace with her death.

As she turned her focus to the person her mother was, the daughter realized that the death was what her mother would have wanted. Knowing the dying person— their beliefs, hopes, and concerns—will help you provide support that addresses and respects their specific needs and wishes.

Providing Support

In the previous pages, I have presented HPC as a resource designed to more fully meet the needs of the dying person and their family. The goal of HPC is to improve the quality of life—the quality of the living and of the dying—for the dying person and the family. PSWs provide physical and psychosocial supports.[8] What can you do to provide support?

Creating a Nurturing Place

Someone once asked me where I wanted to die. Perhaps they were wondering if I wanted to die at home or in the hospital. Immediately I responded, "I want to die in a bed of roses without the thorns." That sounds good to me! A few years later I purchased an outdoor wicker bed with a bright lime green mattress. I told my kids that I had found the bed that I would die on—outside under the stars. I failed to mention that wherever I die, I hope that I get wrapped in lovely warm flannel sheets on a regular basis!

---

8 According to the Canadian Educational Standards for Personal Care Providers related to caring for people with palliative and end of life needs, the PSW "provides emotional support for the client and his/her family."

Carl Rogers, a well-known psychologist, did not mention the outdoor bed or the bed of roses, but he suggested that if we nurture, and are warm, accepting and real, the natural capacity for healing within the person can expand and grow. Developing the following good communication practices are essential to supporting the person's capacity to heal.

Being real

When I read what Carl Rogers wrote about realness, I think of the story of *The Velveteen Rabbit*,[9] a delightful children's book by Margery Williams:

> *"What is REAL?" asked the Rabbit one day, when they were lying side by side near the nursery fender, before Nana came to tidy the room. "Does it mean having things that buzz inside you and a stick-out handle?"*
>
> *"Real isn't how you are made," said the Skin Horse. "It's a thing that happens to you. When a child loves you for a long, long time, not just to play with, but REALLY loves you, then you become Real."*
>
> *"Does it hurt?" asked the Rabbit.*
>
> *"Sometimes," said the Skin Horse, for he was always truthful. "When you are Real you don't mind being hurt."*
>
> *"Does it happen all at once, like being wound up," he asked, "or bit by bit?"*
>
> *"It doesn't happen all at once," said the Skin Horse. "You become. It takes a long time. That's why it doesn't happen often to people who break easily, or have sharp edges, or who have to be carefully kept. Generally, by the time you are Real, most of your hair has been loved off, and your eyes drop out and you get loose in the joints and very shabby. But these things don't matter at all, because once you are Real you can't be ugly, except to people who don't understand."*

I think of the many PSWs I have met over the years, whose hair has not been loved off and whose eyes have not dropped out, but whose presence was real and genuine.

Expressing empathy

Empathy is the ability to understand a person's experience, and what the experience means for that person. Empathy opens the door to conversation. When one person expresses empathy, the focus is on trying to understand the other person, learning what the other person's needs are and finding out how to support the person.

Avoiding roadblocks

There are a few roadblocks that block empathy and therefore block communication, and a few traps that prevent you from being supportive. The roadblocks include minimizing the problem, offering false reassurance, offering sympathy, attempting to fix the problem, and judging and labelling the person.

---

9 M. Williams, *The Velveteen Rabbit*, http://digital.library.upenn.edu/women/williams/rabbit/rabbit. html.

Minimizing the problem

When you get a parking ticket, it may be good to have someone remind you that you could have worse problems. Comments such as "It could be worse" or "My friend got a parking ticket and a speeding ticket on the same day" may make you smile and acknowledge your good fortune. But when a person is dying, efforts to minimize their problems are more likely to leave the person feeling that they have not been heard or understood.

Offering false reassurance

When a person is constipated, it may be helpful when the caregiver assures them that the medication will resolve the problem, but when a person is dying, offering simple statements such as "Everything is going to be just fine" is not helpful and does not address the deep worries and anxieties the person is experiencing.

Offering praise

When a person is facing death and/or the loss of a loved one, receiving praise may feel good in the moment. If you repeatedly praise the person for being strong, resilient, and resourceful, however, they may not want to share or acknowledge their feelings or ask for help when they feel weak, fragile, or lost.

Offering platitudes

Platitudes are trite and shallow statements. Comments such as "Time will heal all wounds" or "The grief will pass" are not true. Time does not heal, and grief does not simply pass. The truth, told with compassion, is helpful to a dying person.

Offering sympathy

One dictionary defines "sympathy" as "the act or capacity of entering into or sharing the feelings or interests of another."[10] This definition suggests a meaning similar to that of "empathy," which may be defined as "the ability to understand another person's experience." Being present and listening to another person expressing their feelings opens the door to communication and connection with that person.

Some people believe that those who display sympathy are more focused on themselves than on the person with whom they are sympathizing. For example, Person A hears that Person B's mother just died and says, "I feel just horrible that your mom died." In that sentence, Person A appears to be more focused on himself than on Person B. Or Person A might say, "That must be hard. My mother died as well, and it was really hard for me. And it is still hard." Again, Person A appears to be focused on himself and does not acknowledge of how Person B feels.

Empathy is not the same as sympathy.

---

10 Merriam-Webster online dictionary, http://www.merriam-webster.com/dictionary/sympathy.

> **Empathy versus Sympathy**
>
> Sympathy is about talking: "I am sorry for you."
>
> Empathy is about listening: "It sounds like this is really hard for you. I want to understand how this is for you. Can you tell me more?"
>
> Sympathy is about standing apart: "Please accept my condolences."
>
> Empathy is about being with: "I am here for you. Please tell me what would be helpful."
>
> Sympathy is often about offering false reassurance: "You will be just fine; everything will turn out all right."
>
> Empathy is about acknowledging uncertainties: "Living with so much uncertainty must be difficult."

Differences between empathy and sympathy

Some people use the word "sympathy" to refer to what others might term "empathy," and others use "sympathy" in the more self-focused sense described above. The use of the words may be less important than the type of message being communicated. Empathy opens the door to communication. Sympathy shuts that door. An empathic (or "empathetic") response focuses on trying to understand another person's feelings and needs. Empathy is about getting close to and connecting with another person.

Compassion is empathy combined with a desire to help.

Getting caught in the Fix-It Trap

If you like to fix problems, and if you think it is your job to fix things, then you may fall into the "Fix-It Trap." When you work with people who are dying, every day you work in the face of unfixable pain and suffering. You cannot fix deep emotional and spiritual pains. That is impossible.

You cannot fix deep emotional and spiritual pain.

Additionally, when you think it is your job to fix things—when you think that a good PSW is one who "fixes"—then you may see, hear, and focus only on problems that you can fix. You may ask to be assigned to people with "simple" problems and avoid people whose issues are complex.

Remember, your job is to support. It is not your job to fix.

Judging and labelling people

When you try to fix but are unable to fix, you might find yourself judging and labelling people. You may judge and label as "good" those families that appear to be less complicated and less demanding, and more compliant, agreeable, appreciative, and, of course, more patient. You may judge and label as "difficult" those families that ask a lot of questions, are strong advocates for their dying loved one, express their grief and stress in unique ways, and/or struggle with complex relationships and unresolved issues.

When people who work in the health care field refer to the "difficult dying person" or the "difficult family member," they usually mean someone who is uncooperative, non-compliant, aggressive, or ungrateful.

Labels and judgements prevent you from seeing the person and their needs

Labels are not helpful; they do not identify the problems and do not describe best strategies to support the person. Labelling someone as "difficult" is a judgment, one that destroys curiosity and stops you from wanting to know more about the person, and from trying to understand who they are and what they need.

Rather than labelling a person as "difficult," it may be more helpful to think of "difficult situations" in which you do your best to work with the people you care for to make things easier for everyone.

Offering a compassionate presence

When you work with the dying, you are in the presence of suffering. Their issues are often complex. Cure is not an option. Death is on the horizon. What does support and compassion look like when the person you care for is in the depths of despair?

Henri Nouwen, a Catholic priest, as well as a professor and writer, wrote this about compassion:

> Let us not underestimate how hard it is to be compassionate. Compassion is hard because it requires the inner disposition to go with others to the place where they are weak, vulnerable, lonely and broken. But it is not our spontaneous response to suffering. What we desire most is to do away with suffering by fleeing from it or finding a quick cure for it … And so we ignore our greatest gift, which is our ability to enter into solidarity with those who suffer.[11]

When working with people in a crisis you need to "...feel your way moment by moment..."

Stephen Levine, a poet, author, and teacher best known for his books on dying, once said that working with people in crisis is similar to reading Braille: you need to feel your way moment by moment. And so it is that you, as a PSW, need to put aside your own agenda and be with the dying person—breathe, sit, and feel your way moment by moment.

I sometimes joke that the most important thing we can learn to say is *nothing*, and the most difficult thing we can learn to do is *nothing*. I am reminded that we are "human beings" not "human doings," and that "being" and "being still" are often as effective as or more effective than "doing." Sitting still and breathing with a dying person may be one of the most effective ways to provide support and care.

---

11 H. Nouwen, *The Way of the Heart: Desert Spirituality and Contemporary Ministry* (New York: Seabury Press, 1981), 34.

I saw her standing, alone and crying, at the back of the room. I did not know her. I did not know why she was crying. I did not know what to say or what to do. I went to her side. I stood next to her. I thought to put my arm around her to communicate caring. I wanted to be supportive, to be helpful. I had no idea what she might find helpful. I stood silently, and eventually I thought to breathe. Slow, deep, breaths. One after another. Deep enough that she would feel them through our physical contact. After a while she stopped crying. She turned to me, opened her phone, and showed me the word she had programmed to come to life when she opened the phone: "BREATHE."

You can be a compassionate presence in a dying person's journey without having to do or say something to fill up the space. When you are present, you are inviting the person to be present as well. And in this gentle safe place you have created, the person may observe their suffering, fear, pain, and confusion in a different way.

Supportive care is being a compassionate presence

To "be there" for someone who is in a difficult situation, stop for a moment. Pay attention to the natural rhythm of your breathing. Notice that you inhale, exhale, pause, inhale, exhale, pause. The silent pause is as much a part of the natural breathing pattern as the inhaling and exhaling. If you skip the pause, you will be hyperventilating, which is an abnormal breathing pattern that cannot be sustained over a long period of time.

In a similar way, communication patterns that are natural include times of pausing and moments of silence. Yet people are often uncomfortable in shared silent moments and, as a result, either avoid or interrupt them. Many people associate silence with emptiness or absence, when in fact silence is full of presence: there is always something going on in the spaces between one's words and actions. Embracing present silence is a conscious clearing of space, a making room for whatever needs to happen. Present silence requires some degree of trust—in yourself, in the other person, or of the situation itself. Present silence requires that you give up controlling the space long enough to allow something to happen (something that the other person directs).

Supportive care makes room for present silence

Present silence can be a gift that allows the dying and the grieving time to collect their thoughts, to face their challenges, and to regroup.

Present silence can be a gift for those who struggle to think and who benefit from the time to ponder and prepare their thoughts.

Present silence can be a gift for those who are fatigued; the space may provide them time to gather the energy to speak.

Good communication is often seen as a skill, but supportive, compassionate communication that includes present silence is an art.

When I was a child, I was taught that in order to be safe when crossing the street I needed to stop, look, and listen. Stop, look both ways, and listen for oncoming cars. As a young hospice nurse, I realized this wisdom applied when caring for a dying person and their family. When I stop, I put my agenda and needs on hold. When I look, I look at the person, their physical presence, their surroundings, their family. When I listen, I listen to what is being said and consider what might be felt but not said. If I stop, look, and listen, then sometimes I am invited to cross the street and journey with the dying person. At some point, the person moves forward alone on their journey, and I remain behind. My life is changed. And sometimes I feel that I have been taught by "the masters."

Compassionate support is about being present in the face of unfixable pain: When you provide such support, you are saying, "I can see the pain in your eyes and hear the pain and worry in your voice. I am here with you."

Supporting dignity

Supportive care includes supporting dignity

How people who are receiving help from the health care system see themselves is affected by how they think other people see them.[12] Wow! That means that how you communicate caring to the person will affect how they see themselves even when you are not with them. You, as a PSW, can have a strong impact on the dignity of those you care for. You are like a mirror that the person and their family use to judge their status in the system. Dr. Harvey Chochinov, a psychiatrist and HPC physician, discovered that dignity is the most important indicator of a person's experience of well-being.

Dignity is the most important indicator of well being

Dr. Chochinov and his team developed a list of questions to ask dying people that would help caregivers identify what they could do to provide the best care possible. Eventually, he and his team were able to identify the one most important question, the one question that would give *the* most important information to help caregivers identify how to best provide care. The "dignity question" is this:

The Dignity Question

What do I need to know about you as a person to give you the best care possible?

Research has shown that this one single question can help you identify important issues to consider when caring for a dying person. This question may help reveal what might not otherwise be discovered. The person's answers to this question will take you behind your assumptions, past your baggage and beliefs, so that you can attend to the needs of the person. This question will help you address the person's very personal needs, hopes, fears, and anxieties.

You can ask this question when someone is first admitted to care, and again as care progresses. You may consider and ponder this question privately or in conversation with the family when you work with someone who is not able to or does not like

---

12 Dignity in Care, http://dignityincare.ca/en/toolkit.html#The_Patient_Dignity_Question.

to communicate verbally. Asking the dignity question can help you identify and attend to the needs and wishes of the dying person.

Samples of Dignity Questions

"What do I need to know about you as a person to give you the best care possible?"

"Well … I hate pain, I like answers to my questions, and I like people who care for me to be warm and friendly."

"Okay. So, how about we enjoy our time together when I come, and I make sure you are comfortable before I provide care, and if you have questions that are not being answered, I will write a note for the nurse to speak with you?"

"That's good, dear."

"What do I need to know about you as a person to give you the best care possible?"

"Well, first of all I don't want help. It is hard for me to need care. But when I really have to have help, then I want care to be excellent and to have people arrive on time. I do not want a bunch of different people who don't know me or the routine. I want them to know what they are doing. And once that happens, then I like to talk with everyone I meet."

"So, you don't like to need care, but if you are going to have it, you want it to be excellent, on time, provided by consistent people, and when good care is provided, then you want to enjoy talking with those who provide your care."

"Yes, you have understood me perfectly!"

"What do I need to know about you as a person to give you the best care possible?"

"I don't like asking for help, so people need to be aware and do what is needed and be on their way."

"Okay, so we need to make sure that we outline the tasks so that people will know what to do."

"Yes, I don't like a lot of questions and chatter."

Communicating

Dorothee Soelle, in her book *Suffering*, states that people need to speak of their affliction or they will be swallowed up in it. She suggests that it does not matter whether they communicate verbally or nonverbally, but they need to express themselves. She states, "People's lives actually depend on … learning to express themselves, which includes the nonverbal possibilities of expression. Without the capacity to communicate, there can be no change."[13]

To help people grow in a safe place, you can open the door to invite expression.

Open the door for people to express themselves

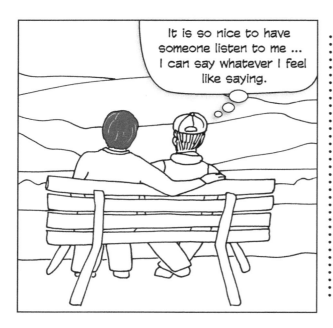
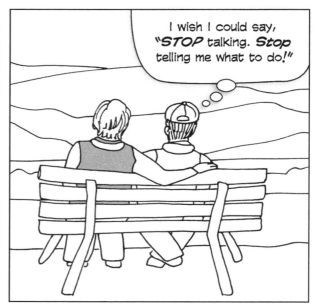

13 D. Soelle, *Suffering* (Philadelphia: Fortress Press, 1975), 76.

Asking open-ended questions

As a PSW, you can create a space where a dying person feels safe, where the door is open to exploration, and where nurturing ground can foster growth. When you ask open-ended questions, you can gather information and understand the person's needs and preferences for psychosocial support and physical comfort measures. Open-ended questions may also help the person reflect on and explore their own experience. When you ask open-ended questions, you allow the person to feel seen and heard and understood.

Benefits of asking open-ended questions

Here are some examples of open-ended questions:

Hmm ... can you tell me more?

What do you think?

What is happening?

Can you give me an example?

What do you need right now in order to feel safe?

What do we need to know about you to provide the best care possible?

"Can you tell me more?" is an open-ended question

Open-ended questions are elements of good communication because they have the following effects:
- Encourage conversation
- Help the dying person share their story
- Allow you to see and hear the person
- Help the person feel heard without feeling judged
- Help you communicate and validate the person's experiences
- Help prevent misunderstandings

Sometimes it is helpful to clarify what the person is saying:

I wonder if what you're saying is ...?

So, I get the sense that ... Is that right?

Responding reflectively may bring clarity to the person

A non-judgemental, reflective response can help the person further explore their experience and help you gain clarity and understanding.

When someone is dying, people often hope for, wish for, pray for a cure and for "healing." There is a difference between curing and healing. Curing may be defined as fixing or solving the problem that is causing the illness. Healing, on the other hand, is a more internal, psychosocial process, an inner feeling of wholeness. Rachel Naomi Remen, a pioneer in the field of mind-body health, suggests that people are healed when they are seen and heard and validated.

It is interesting to me that seeing, hearing, and validating are all a part of providing compassionate support.

When you observe and listen with respect for the dying person, you can participate in healing.

People heal when they
are heard, seen and
validated.

The Team at Base Camp

John Amatt, a mountaineer, was the principal organizer and leader of the first team that climbed Mount Everest. He spoke in Victoria, BC, many years ago, and stated that the only reason the team was able to reach the summit of the mountain was because of the supporting team at the base camp.

In HPC, the health care team provides the support at the "base camp." The team includes you, the PSW! You care, support, connect, communicate, and advocate for and on behalf of the dying person and their family. You create a safe place for them when you are genuine, express empathy, open the door to communication, provide a compassionate presence, and are comfortable with silence. You support the dignity of the dying person and can best meet their needs when you ask,

What do I need to know about you to provide the best care possible?

PSWs support the
person and family to
grow and live as fully as
possible

And, in this safe, nurturing, supportive place that you help create, the dying person and their family are more able to grow during their suffering and live as fully as possible through the process of dying and grieving.

The Story of Martha

I arrived at the home to pronounce the death of the mother, help prepare her body, and provide support for the family. The PSW served tea to the woman's husband and settled him in his large recliner. She then sat with the woman's daughter and listened to stories of her mother and of growing up on the prairies.

After I completed my tasks, we visited while we waited for the funeral home attendants to arrive. The daughter talked of the care received from the health care team and the benefits of having a PSW. She said, "Everyone was helpful, the nurses, the doctors, the counsellor, the neighbours, the cancer agency … but Martha, the PSW, she made it all work. She has been here 24 hours a day. She listened to each of us, she listened to my brothers, she listened to me, and she talked with my dad and my mom. She knew how to listen. She did not offer advice except when we specifically asked her to. Martha gave my mom excellent physical care. Martha knew what to expect. When we got worried about some change with Mom, Martha knew when to call for help, and she knew when to tell us not to worry. When Mom's breathing became irregular, Martha told us this was normal. A while later, when the breathing sounds became wet, Martha told us that we needed to call the home care nurse. Martha made the whole thing work."

Before I left the home, I pulled Martha aside and asked her how she developed such competence in caregiving. Martha described the support she received from the nurse supervisor at her agency; she talked about the home care nurses who provided expert care and involved her in their assessments, answered her questions, and modelled excellent care. Martha also told of the education that she had received in a workshop on caring for the dying.

Not all deaths are this peaceful, not all teams function this well, and not all people are able to access 24-hour home support services in the last few days. Nevertheless, I left this home contemplating the benefits of good teamwork, the participation of each individual to influence the overall care, and the impact of a great PSW!

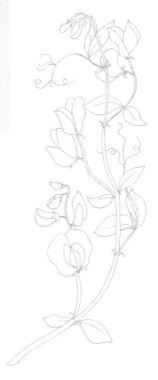

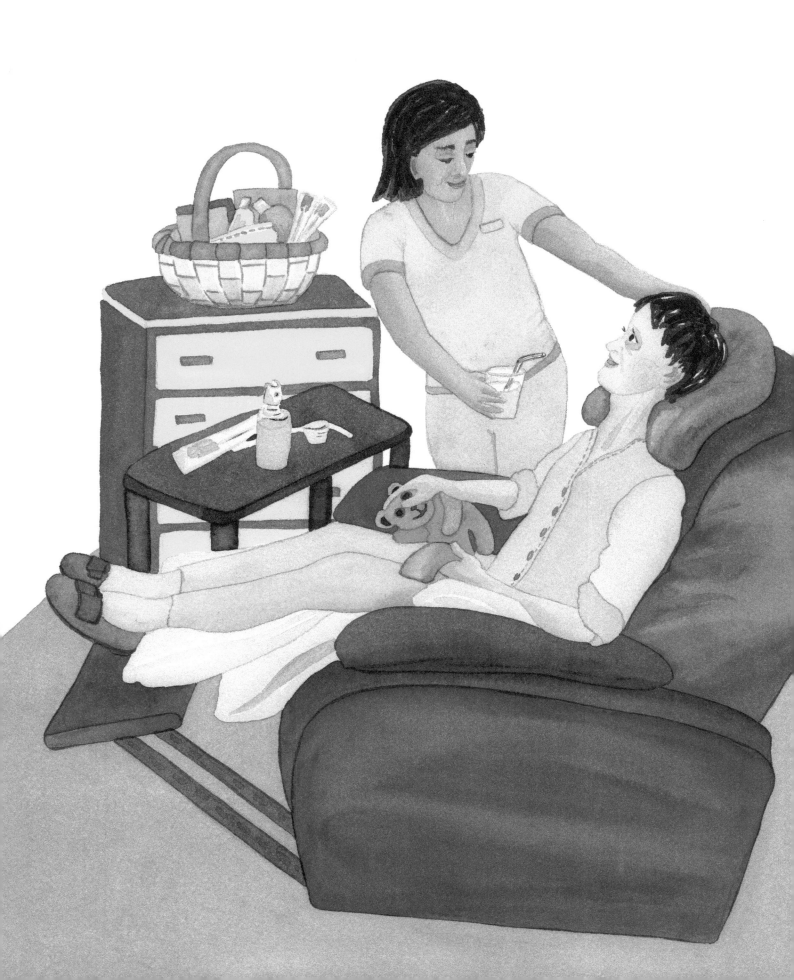

Increasing Physical Comfort

Part 1: Tools, Communication, and Palliation

I have heard people say, "It is not being dead but the dying I fear." People often fear the physical suffering associated with dying. The focus of Part 1 of this chapter is to provide PSWs with a few key tools—the Palliative Performance Scale and the List of Sample Questions—and tips on recording (documenting), reporting, and advocating that will help you gather information about the person and communicate it to the health care team. The chapter also reviews the principles of palliation and the use of medications to help manage common symptoms. The dying person, their family, and formal caregivers often have concerns about the use of opioids, so that topic is addressed in detail. A discussion of nonpharmacological measures to provide comfort follows. Finally, in Part 2, the chapter elaborates on each of nine common symptoms you may observe in the dying person.

People often fear the physical suffering associated with dying

Tools for Gathering Information

Can you look after Mr. K.? He was 60% last week, 40% yesterday, and is 20% today. The family is blown away and needs support.

You may not understand what this statement means … unless you speak the language of the Victoria Hospice Palliative Performance Scale (PPS).[1] You will be using the PPS and the List of Sample Questions[2] to gather and share information about the dying person's needs. The List of Sample Questions is adapted from a tool specifically designed to support the gathering of information required for effective symptom management. Understanding the terminology and tools used in hospice palliative care (HPC) will help you communicate more clearly and easily. As you become more comfortable with the List of Sample Questions, you will be able to adapt the questions to gather important information about any symptom. When

Gather information with the PPS and List of Sample Questions

Using these tools may get a more timely and appropriate response from the nurse

---

1   Victoria Hospice, Palliative Performance Scale. See Appendix C.

2   The List of Sample Questions is adapted from Fraser Health's Symptom Assessment Acronym—OPQRSTUV—which prompts the user to ask comprehensive questions that will help the user to complete a thorough assessment and thus improve symptom management. To simplify the list of questions and make it more accessible for PSWs, the acronym is not provided in this text but is available from http://www.fraserhealth.ca/media/SymptomAssessmentRevised_Sept09.pdf.

you provide that information to the appropriate health care professional,[3] it will help them decide how best to respond. When you provide a clear report you are more likely to get a timely and appropriate response from the nurse.

The Victoria Hospice Palliative Performance Scale

PPS gathers information on the person's level of functioning

The PPS is a tool for gathering information on key indicators and behaviours that will help the members of the care team understand the level of functioning and declining condition of the person for whom they are caring.

PPS levels decrease with dying

This tool describes a person's level of functioning on a percentage scale, from 100%, which indicates that the person is disease-free and completely functional, to 0%, meaning death. The person's mobility level (ambulation), activity level and evidence of disease, ability for self-care, intake, and level of consciousness are observed and assigned a percentage value.

Changes in each of these areas are common throughout the dying process. Observing how the person behaves in each area will help the nurse understand their needs, declining condition, and rate of change. The PPS also serves as an excellent communication tool, providing a quick summary and status update on the person.

PPS identifies changes in key indicators of the dying process

Use of the PPS facilitates knowledge sharing, communication of the person's needs, and care planning by revealing changes in key indicators of the dying process. It can also be helpful in determining how long a person has to live.

Using the PPS

The PPS is used across Canada in the community and in hospice and palliative care settings, and is increasingly being used in long-term care and acute care settings. You can use the PPS as a framework to guide your observations and what you report each day. As the days and weeks pass, you may notice daily changes and realize that the person is changing and declining quickly. Or you may notice that the person is the same day after day, in which case you will need to report only if a change occurs.

Use the PPS to help you report on
• ambulation
• activity level
• self-care
• intake
• consciousness

As you look at the PPS table on the next page, consider how you might comment on each of the following indicators to provide valuable information:
- Ambulation: Is the person fully mobile, or is their mobility reduced? For example, is the person mainly sitting and lying, mainly in bed, or totally bed bound?
- Activity level: Is the person able to do their normal job or work, unable to do any work, unable to do most activities, or unable to do any activities?

---

3 The PSW works under the direction of a health care professional. This is often a nurse. In this text, "nurse" refers to the person the PSW reports to.

- Self-care: Is the person able to do their own self-care, or does the person require occasional assistance, considerable assistance, assistance with most things, or total care?
- Intake: Is the person's intake normal, reduced, or minimal (only sips), or does the person receive only mouth care?
- Consciousness level or mentation: Is the person fully alert and conscious? Does the person have some confusion, or is the person drowsy at times, drowsy but fully conscious at times, or in a coma?

Samples of records (documentation) and reports (often given to the nurse orally) are included throughout the text to assist you in preparing your records and reports.

Sample Report

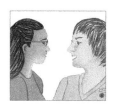

❝ I am with Mr. M. He is totally bed bound, is unable to do any of his normal activities, requires total care, is taking only sips of fluids, and is drowsy and awake for only short periods. ❞

Sample PPS report

Victoria Hospice

Palliative Performance Scale (PPSv2) version 2

PPS Level	Ambulation	Activity & Evidence of Disease	Self-Care	Intake	Conscious Level
100%	Full	Normal activity & work No evidence of disease	Full	Normal	Full
90%	Full	Normal activity & work Some evidence of disease	Full	Normal	Full
80%	Full	Normal activity with effort Some evidence of disease	Full	Normal or reduced	Full
70%	Reduced	Unable normal job/work Significant disease	Full	Normal or reduced	Full
60%	Reduced	Unable hobby/house work Significant disease	Occasional assistance necessary	Normal or reduced	Full or Confusion
50%	Mainly Sit/Lie	Unable to do any work Extensive disease	Considerable assistance required	Normal or reduced	Full or Confusion
40%	Mainly in Bed	Unable to do most activity Extensive disease	Mainly assistance	Normal or reduced	Full or Drowsy +/– Confusion
30%	Totally Bed Bound	Unable to do any activity Extensive disease	Total Care	Normal or reduced	Full or Drowsy +/– Confusion
20%	Totally Bed Bound	Unable to do any activity Extensive disease	Total Care	Minimal to sips	Full or Drowsy +/– Confusion
10%	Totally Bed Bound	Unable to do any activity Extensive disease	Total Care	Mouth care only	Drowsy or Coma +/– Confusion
0%	Death	—	—	—	—

Reproduced with permission. Copyright Victoria Hospice Society, BC, Canada (2001), .

The List of Sample Questions

The List of Sample Questions will help PSWs gather information about specific symptoms. This act of gathering information will assure the dying person and their family that you are attending to the person's needs. The information you gather will help you and the health care team adapt the care plan according to the person's needs and individualize the comfort measures you provide. When you communicate this information, it will help the nurse understand the needs of the person and family and respond in an appropriate, timely way.

The questions in the list below are only sample questions. Rephrase and adapt them to address the specific symptoms you encounter.

Modify sample questions to address specific symptoms

Adapt sample questions to suit each person's communication needs.

- What is happening? What is wrong?
- When did it start?
- Where do you feel it?
- How does it feel?
- Can you rate it on a scale?
  - 0 to 10 (0 = no symptom and 10 = the worst imaginable)
  - Small, medium, large
  - Mild, moderate, severe
- What makes it better or worse?
- What would be helpful? What can I do to help you?
- What do you want to see/have happen?

Before asking the dying person and their family questions like those in the List of Sample Questions, consider the following to help you decide what questions would be helpful to ask right now:

- Consider how the person and their family are managing the volume of questions they are asked, the number of people who are involved in providing care, and whether the person and family are struggling to repeat information to various members of the team. If the person and family are overwhelmed with too many questions from too many people, it may be best to let the nurse gather all the information at one time. On the other hand, if the dying person is feeling that care is lacking or that no one has asked or cares about their concerns, they may find it very helpful to have you ask questions, record the information, and report the information you gather to the nurse. If a new symptom has appeared or a symptom has increased in severity, the person may be anxious to see the nurse or the doctor and may especially appreciate you asking about the symptom and reporting it.
- Consider what you need to know in order to provide the best care for this person. What do you need to know before moving ahead with the scheduled care for the visit? If the person is in severe pain, you may need to postpone the bath and focus on providing comfort measures, communicating with the team, and reorganizing the day.
- Consider how you can personalize care. What do you need to know to personalize the comfort measures? Do you already know that a warm cloth and a foot rub help this person relax until their medication takes effect? You might

need to ask either the person or the family what you can do to help or provide comfort.

- Consider what the health care team requires in order to move ahead and provide good care. What information do you need to provide to help the nurse understand what is happening for this person and respond in a timely and helpful way? If the nurse is nearby, is familiar with the person, and is able to respond in minutes, then you may not need to ask the person many questions. If, on the other hand, the nurse is not nearby, does not know the person, does not know their history, and is not familiar with how they express pain or how they best communicate, it may be helpful for you to gather the relevant information and try to help the nurse understand what is happening.

What information is needed to respond in a timely and helpful way?

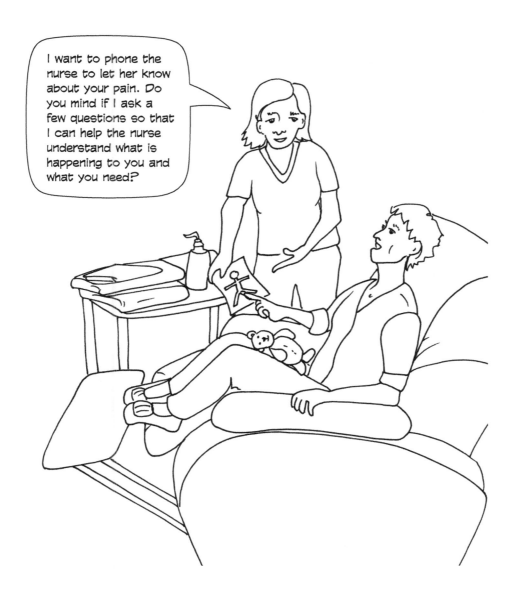

Communicating with the Team

Sometimes I hear the PSW say, "The practical nurse doesn't listen to me."

And sometimes I hear the practical nurse say, "The RN doesn't listen to me."

And sometimes I hear the nurses say, "The physician doesn't listen to me."

And sometimes I hear the person and family say, "No one listens to me!"

Clear, concise recording and reporting will help you to be heard by the team

If you do not record and report in a clear, concise way, you may not be heard. If your record and report are clear, concise, and easy to understand, you are more likely to see people respond in an appropriate, timely way.

Recording and Reporting

As a PSW, you need to follow agency or facility policies for documentation. Here are some tips on recording (documenting) and reporting that might be helpful to you.

Tips for clear, concise recording and reporting

When you record and report,
- Write the information so it is clear to someone who was not there
- Do not write assumptions and value judgments
- Keep records brief and to the point
- Provide only necessary information

When recording,
- State whom (which nurse) you reported to
- Use correct grammar and spelling
- Sign your documentation

When reporting, if you ask for assistance, make clear what you are asking the nurse to do.

When you prepare a report to give to the nurse or at a care conference, organize your thoughts in advance. If you have a history of not being heard, practise delivering the report to a colleague in advance.

What to include in an excellent report

When you report, remembering to include the following will help you provide an excellent report:
- Give the person's name and the time of your visit/interaction.
- If the nurse does not know the person, provide a background summary and PPS.
- Identify the concern you are contacting the nurse about.
- Summarize the information you gathered when you adapted the List of Sample Questions.

- Identify the comfort measures that either you or other members of the health care team provided.
- Identify any other symptoms or changes in the patient, such as decreased level of consciousness.
- State clearly your request.

Sample Record

●●● June 4, 2014, 0830. I attempted to help Helene sit up this morning. Helene called out in pain, pushed my hand away, held the right side of her abdomen, was unable to move her legs off the bed with assistance. No previous reports of pain. This is a change in her behaviour. Helene unable to answer any questions regarding pain. Settled on her left side. Warm blanket provided. Quiet moaning at rest. On-call nurse (Yoshi S.) notified and asked to assess Helene. ●●●

Sample Record indicating changes in the person's pain and behaviour

Sample Report

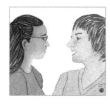

❝ I want to talk with you about Helene W. I just went to provide her morning care. Normally she is able to sit up, move to the side of the bed, transfer to her wheelchair. Today she called out in pain when I attempted to help her sit up and move her to the side of the bed. She pushed my hand away. She is holding the right side of her abdomen. She is not able to report where her pain is, or answer any questions about the pain. The night staff had not reported any concerns. This is a major change in her behaviour. I settled her on her left side, and gave her a warm blanket. She is lying still but moaning quietly at rest.

Can you come and see her? ❞

Sample Report to Nurse

Sample Record

●●● Jag has an increase in pain in his right hip. It started this morning. It hurts from his right hip down the right leg. He rates pain at 3/10. His wife says that he is strong and does not like to talk about pain. She rates his pain at 6/10. Jag feels a bit better when I put a pillow under his right leg and wrap a warm flannel across him and down his leg. He wants to see the nurse or doctor. ●●●

Sample Record indicating changes in a person's pain

Sample Report

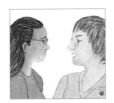

❝ *Jag has an increase in pain, right hip. It started this morning. It hurts from his right hip down the right leg. He rates pain at 3/10. His wife says that he is strong and does not like to talk about pain. She rates his pain at 6/10. Jag feels a bit better when I put a pillow under his right leg and wrap a warm flannel across his him and down his leg. He wants to see the nurse or doctor. What should I do about his morning care? I was supposed to bathe him this morning.* ❞

Advocating

An advocate is a person who pleads for or on behalf of another person, and to advocate is to speak or write in favour of another person. As a PSW, you advocate on behalf of the person and their family, and you help them advocate for themselves.

Ways to advocate

Lynelle Hamilton, an educator and the director of the PSW Educational Program Accreditation agency in Ontario, suggests that in your role as a PSW you are an advocate when you

- Clarify information to clear up misconceptions

  Here is the brochure outlining the services. I think it will help you understand what is available.

- Connect the person or family with someone who can assist

  Can I suggest that you speak with the nurse, or talk with the director of care about extra services that are available?

- Connect the person or family with a health care provider when they need to advocate for themselves

  You sound very concerned that your husband is not receiving the pain medication and the support that he requires to be comfortable. These are important concerns to share. Have you thought about talking with the nurse, the director of care, or your husband's doctor?

  You are very clear that you do not want to die in pain. Have you talked with the nurse about this? Can I mention to the nurse how important this is to you? Are there other things that you want to make sure the nurse or health care team knows about?

Advocating includes
- **clarifying**
- **connecting with resources**
- **identifying information and concerns that need to be shared with the health care team**

- Identify information that the person or family will need to present in order to advocate for themselves

  When you talk with the nurse or the doctor, it will be important to share your observations, what your husband would have said or wanted if he was able to speak for himself, and the goals or focus of care. Here are the phone numbers if you need them.

Tips on advocating

You may need to advocate when the dying person's condition changes and when physical or psychosocial issues arise. You need to advocate on the phone if you work in the community, one to one in a facility, and to the care team in care conferences. In each of these settings, there are times when it may be more difficult to advocate. Here are some tips to help you prepare and present your concerns when you advocate to the nurse, health care team, and/or family:

Ways to boost your success at advocating

- Be confident.
- Be professional.
- Be prepared (follow suggestions above for recording and reporting).
- Be clear.
- Be descriptive and avoid making conclusions.
- Be positive and express gratitude for support offered—assume that everyone wants what is best for the dying person.

Remember that the less the nurse is involved with and knows about the person, the better your report will need to be. The sample reports below illustrate both poor and good reporting.

Reports must be *more* thorough when the nurse is *less* involved

Sample Reports

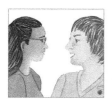

[Poor] 66 ~~Ellen needs more pain medication.~~ 99

[Good] 66 *For the past three days, Ellen has needed breakthrough doses every day. She says her pain is increasing. Previously, she said she was comfortable until the next dose was given. Now she says that she is comfortable for only a few hours.* 99

Comparison of a good and bad report

You can use these tips for advocating on behalf of the dying person when you are addressing visiting neighbours, friends, or extended family. Sometimes the person or immediate family will want you to help be the "gate keeper" and decrease the number of people visiting, the number of visits, or the length of visits. In that case, and with the permission of the person or the family, you can tape a note to the person's door that states a clear, simple, and positive message about visiting.

> **Visitors**
>
> Josef loves visitors but tires easily. Please limit visits to 5 minutes.

Palliation

Principles of Palliation

Principles for comfort management

These principles guide the health care team when managing symptoms of the dying person in HPC:

- Focus on person's goals of care.
- Remember that information and education help the person and the family participate in symptom management.
- Prevent symptoms that can be prevented.
- Individualize comfort measures and use nonpharmacological ones when possible.
- Use medications for managing symptoms when necessary.
- Monitor, record, and report the person's responses to medications and other comfort measures.

Principles of Using Medications to Manage Symptoms

These principles guide the ordering and administration of medications:

- The dying person determines the goal for pain relief.
- It is easier to prevent pain than to respond to a pain crisis.
- Medications must be administered regularly, around the clock, to effectively manage ongoing symptoms.
- Breakthrough doses of medication may be needed when a symptom recurs between regularly scheduled doses.
- Generally, it is best to use the simplest delivery route available, usually by mouth. If the person cannot take medications orally, use buccal, rectal, subcutaneous injection, transdermal patch, or topical administration.

Individualize medications to meet the person's goals

- The medication dose should be tailored to meet the person's goals for symptom management while incurring the least side effects possible.
- A combination of medications may be necessary to control a symptom and side effects.
- Side effects and fears or concerns about medications should be recorded and reported.
- Nonpharmacological comfort measures may help improve comfort.
- Responses to medications and comfort measures are an essential part of ongoing assessment and should be recorded and reported.

Follow-up is essential

It is as important to follow-up after medications are given as it is to gather information initially. The response to medications can be determined by asking yourself or the person you are caring for questions like these:

- Did the medication help?
- Was the symptom relieved?
- Is the symptom unchanged?
- Did the symptom increase?

- Did the symptom reoccur before the next dose?
- Did side effects occur?

It is essential that you record and report the dying person's response to medication. Communicate promptly to the health care team any changes in the person's condition, or inability or unwillingness to take medication, and share the person's and the family's concerns with the nurse or physician.

Record and communicate responses and changes to the health care team

> *When I am asked to see a person who is experiencing pain (or any other symptom), I review their chart to gather information about the pain, medications that have been used, and the effectiveness of the medications. The chart usually includes a brief statement about pain. It is especially helpful if the charting also includes when the pain started, the location, what it feels like, the severity of pain, and any comfort measures or medications that have been trialled. It is essential that the response to comfort measures or medications is recorded a few hours later. This information helps me decide what medication and what dose to order for this person.*

Using Opioids to Manage Symptoms

Medications are an important tool to manage symptoms. Opioids[4] are one type of medication that is essential to managing moderate to severe pain, difficult breathing and coughing. As helpful as opioids are in managing these symptoms, the dying person, their family, and members of the health care team often have fears about opioids and their possible side effects and may have difficulty talking about them. If you would like additional information please refer to Appendix A. The side effects of and common fears about opioids are discussed below.[5]

Side effects of opioids

When given opioids, people experience side effects to varying degrees. Constipation may take a few days to develop, while nausea and drowsiness may occur immediately. Some side effects wear off after a few days; for example, drowsiness may last for only 72 hours. Other side effects may continue as long as the person takes the medication.

Addressing the fears about opioids and side effects will help the person and family understand the benefits of opioids

These are some of the common side effects of opioid use:
- Constipation
- Nausea and vomiting
- Confusion and/or delirium
- Drowsiness

---

4 Currently health care professionals use the term "opioids" rather than "narcotics."

5 Additional information on fears about opioids and their side effects is provided in appendix A.

Less common side effects include a dry, sore mouth, itching, urinary retention or hesitancy, and sweating. Too much opioid, over too long a period of time, can result in a buildup of the byproduct of the opioid and cause muscle twitching. Communicate with the nurse if side effects of opioid use occur.

Common fears about opioids

Common fears of opioids:
- side effects
- "I'm dying"
- tolerance
- dependency
- addiction
- respiratory depression

These are the most common fears about opioid use:
- Developing constipation and other side effects
- The implication that a person who is being given opioids must be dying
- Developing tolerance

> *What will happen if he needs more medication because his body gets used to this dose of medication?*

- Becoming dependent

> *What will happen if she gets dependent on the medication?*

- Becoming addicted

> *What will happen if she becomes an addict?*

- Developing respiratory depression

> *What will happen if it slows my breathing down too much?*

For more information about these concerns, see appendix A.

Responding to fears about opioids

If the dying person or their family expresses concerns or has questions about the use of opioids, you might respond,

> *Those are common concerns and good questions. It might be helpful for you to talk with the nurse or physician about this. Can I mention your concerns to them?*

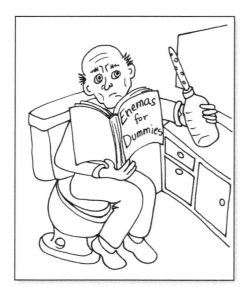
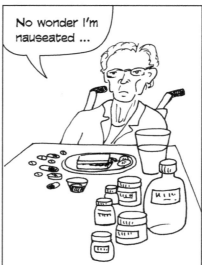
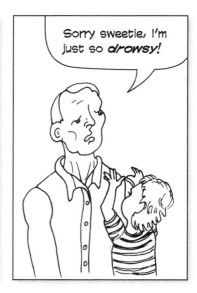

Basket of Comfort Measures— Creativity in Caregiving

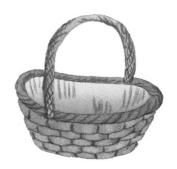

The "comfort basket" is an image I use for the collection of nonpharmaco-logical items PSWs can use to help decrease a dying person's discomfort and provide support. Comfort measures help people relax and may help to distract them from their discomfort. Providing most comfort measures identified in this text does not require a prescription from a doctor, a refer-ral to a specialist, or permission from the nurse. As mentioned elsewhere in this text, it is a good idea for PSWs to check the policies of their agency, facility, or unit to clarify what strategies can be used.

Everyone has their own "basket" of comfort measures that originate from their lives, talents, and other people. Some people sing to comfort, distract, energize, and bring humour to a person who is ill or dying. Other people achieve the same effect by telling funny stories.

Create your own comfort basket

You can also get ideas about what is important to a person by looking on their shelves and walls, and among the things they treasure. For example, in long-term care settings, you may find hand cream on the bathroom counter, pillows in the closet, and a music player on the shelf. If you integrate these items into your care of the person, you are more likely to provide comfort than if you use something from another person's shelves. I remember a woman whose love was music, and she taught the caregivers to arrange different songs to set different moods, depending on her need.

Be creative with comfort measures!

Guidelines for Using the Comfort Basket

It is helpful to keep these guidelines in mind when using the comfort basket:
- Respect the dying person and individualize the care you provide.
- Remember that what works at one point may not work at another.
- Remember that what does not work at one point may work at another.
- Invite the family to participate in providing comfort measures.
- Provide the family with information about the comfort measures you use and how the family can integrate them into caring for the person.
- Encourage the family to think of things the person used to do that brought them comfort. Consider whether those things could be adapted to be com-fort measures now.
- Keep in mind that family members might want to lie next to or snuggle with the person or want time for intimacy. They may want permission to lie on the bed. Side rails can prevent people from falling out of bed. Closing the door can provide some privacy.
- If appropriate, invite family and friends to share their comfort measures.

Individualize comfort measures to the needs of the person at this time

> *I understand that you studied therapeutic touch together. Have you thought of offering a treatment to Bob?*

I hear that you and Sam used to sing together. Would you consider singing for him now?

- Be open to adding new tools to your comfort basket.
- Invite the dying person to teach you new comfort measures.

It is important to choose comfort measures that will best meet the needs and preferences of the person who has a particular symptom at a particular time. The illustration below might inspire you!

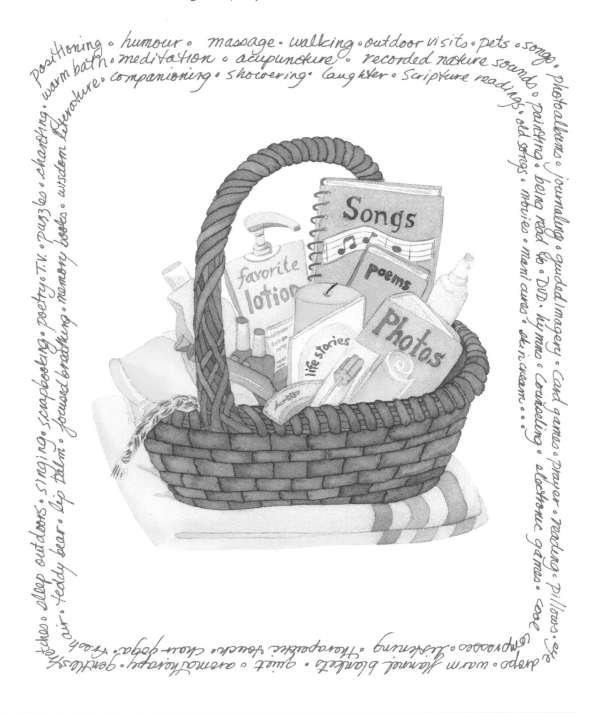

Music Care[6]

The Room 217 Story

When I was growing up, my Sunday afternoon pastime was making music with my dad. He would be at the organ and I would be at the piano. Music drew us together. When Dad had his first and second quadruple bypasses, it was no surprise that music played a role in his recovery. The tunes energized him and gave him hope for recovery.

The diagnosis of stage 4 non-Hodgkins lymphoma was as unexpected as a snowfall in July. I remember one morning in those first months like it was yesterday. He sat in the rocking chair and I sat on his organ bench. Intuitively, we knew our exchange would be about those songs we had played for years. Our tears sang the words that day. Several weeks before Dad died, and just one week before Christmas, I played him familiar carols. These tunes evoked the memories we shared and the hope of one last celebration together. The last hours with Dad are still etched in my heart. In Room 217[6] at the Uxbridge Cottage Hospital, my five siblings, Mom, and I surrounded his bed singing the songs he loved. Dad tried singing along. Music companioned Dad in his final transition. It was a gift, wrapped with the ribbon of release for all of us. —Bev Foster

Music can
- distract
- relax
- spark memories
- increase attention
- facilitate grieving and connecting

Music can improve a person's quality of living, as well as their dying. Carefully chosen music can successfully distract a person from pain, reduce their anxiety or agitation, and promote sleep. Music often holds personal meaning and can connect people to their feelings and memories. For some people, music can improve their ability to attend and remember tasks. Shared songs can also help people grieve, connecting them with others and helping them with the feelings of loss and grief.

---

6 Today, the Room 217 Foundation (http://www.room217.ca), a registered Canadian charity named in my dad's honour, is dedicated to caring for the whole person with music.

Strategies for Adding Music to Caregiving

Gathering Information

Listen to the dying person's environment to decide whether there is room to introduce music into it. Are there other sources of environmental noise (e.g., radio, TV, vacuum, dishwasher)? Is the ambient noise causing discomfort? If so, can you adjust the ambient noise?

When ambient noise creates problems, suggest to the person that using a personal music player with headphones may be helpful.

Ask about the person's musical preferences. Choose music for other people carefully by first asking for their input. A song that brings pleasure to one person could be painful for another. If the person cannot communicate, ask their family. Alternatively, bring in CDs to show the person or play songs and observe the person's responses.

Preparing to Provide Music

Remember to breathe fully and deeply. People convey comfort in the way they breathe and talk. Breathing deeply will ground your speaking voice and make it calming for the person.

Create music while caregiving. Hum or sing softly as you provide care. This builds connections with the person and often creates a feeling of calm and caring. If you do not feel particularly musical, hum a simple song or even a single note. The vibrations from a singer's voice box are calming.

Prepare a music care kit—your personal music care toolbox—to add to your comfort basket. It might include
- A music playing device—mp3 player or CD player or tablet
- Recorded music—selection of music of various genres and speeds

—Bev Foster, Room 217 Foundation

Part 2: Common Symptoms

Changes in Bowel and Bladder Function

This section focuses on the unique challenges presented by bowel and bladder changes that occur when the dying person's mobility and intake decrease, and death is likely in the coming days or weeks.

Constipation is the inability to move the bowels. Although the normal length of time between bowel movements (BMs) varies greatly from person to person, a person is considered to be constipated if they have two or fewer BMs per week. Constipation can be caused by inadequate fluid, inadequate fibre, changes in regular diet or routine, inadequate activity, immobility, medications, lack of good nerve and muscle function, and obstruction due to a tumour. (Many of these causes are common in late-stage disease.)

Causes of constipation

When a person has diarrhea, the large intestine does not absorb water, the stool is liquid, and the person has many loose BMs in a day. Fluid losses with diarrhea can result in dehydration, weakness, and delirium. Causes of diarrhea include medications, therapies such as radiation and chemotherapy, malabsorption of food, surgeries, infections, and some cancers. (Sometimes when a person who is constipated is given laxatives, the softer more liquid stool in a BM bypasses the hard compacted stool.)

Causes of diarrhea

Incontinence is the inability to control the evacuation of urine from the bladder or stool from the bowel. Incontinence is common as a person declines and becomes weaker in the last days and hours. Sometimes incontinence occurs when there is nerve damage; therefore, any sudden changes in urinary control for someone who is not imminently dying should be reported to the nurse. Urinary retention is a side

Causes of incontinence

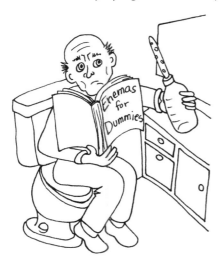

effect that some people experience when taking opioids. Sometimes this is temporary, and normal functioning returns within a few days. Urinary incontinence may result from urinary tract infections, medications, lack of good nerve and muscle function, or weakness. Incontinence can be either temporary or ongoing.

Gathering Information

Observing

PSWs often observe changes in the frequency and/or urgency of the BMs of the person in their care. Such observations should be recorded and reported (e.g., "small amount of hard stool," "straining to have a bowel movement," "small and incomplete movements"), as should the presence of stool in the rectum, oozing liquid stool, stool on pads in undergarments, or soiled undergarments.

Symptoms that may accompany constipation or diarrhea

When a person is constipated or has diarrhea, they may also experience vomiting, nausea, abdominal pain and distention, and generalized pain. Blood, mucus, or pus may be present in stool or urine, it may have a foul odour, and bowel sounds, including flatus, may occur. These symptoms may cause restlessness, agitation, or aggression in the person. If any of these occur, they should be recorded and reported.

Asking questions

Adapting the questions in the List of Sample Questions and asking the person you are caring for your questions will help you understand their needs.

Comfort Measures

Preventive

The person's decreased mobility and intake negatively affect functioning of the bowels and bladder. Maintaining muscle activity when a person's mobility is limited can help prevent problems. Chair exercises that use abdominal muscles and move the legs will help encourage intestinal mobility. When overall dietary intake decreases, insoluble fibre can be incorporated into the person's intake if they are still taking sufficient fluids. Providing a commode near the bed is important when the person's energy or mobility is limited or if urgency becomes an issue.

In the moment

Supporting a person with constipation or diarrhea

These are some ways you can provide comfort:
- Answer call bells as soon as possible.
- Provide privacy measures for the dying person, such as curtains and background noise (e.g., a tap running).
- Provide easy access to toileting facilities.
- Remove and clean the commode immediately after use.
- Assist the person in moving to and from the commode and help them clean up when necessary.
- Protect the skin from irritation when the person is incontinent.
- Consider using a catheter or incontinence pads for a person with urinary incontinence.
- Report a sudden onset of diarrhea or incontinence immediately.

For the family

If family members want to be involved in caregiving, you can show them some things they can do to help:

- Arrange the room so the dying person has sufficient privacy when using the commode.
- Communicate the person's questions to the health care team.
- Record (document) the date and quality of the person's BMs, including a description.

Medications and Treatments

Administering medications regularly can prevent or treat constipation and diarrhea. A combination of medications may be needed. Dosages and the duration of treatment will depend on the cause of the problem and the goals of care. If oral medication does not relieve the symptom, a suppository or enema may be required.

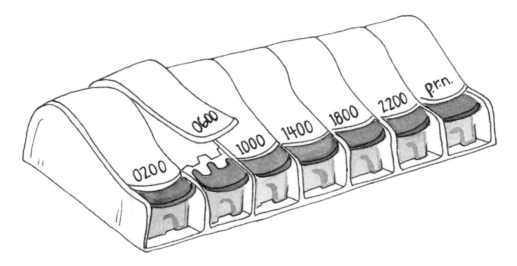

Decreased Appetite and Weight Loss

Please tell my wife not to bring me so much food. It makes me sick just looking at it!

Please tell my husband to eat more food. If he doesn't eat, he will die.

Loss of appetite and weight commonly occur as disease progresses

The appetite commonly decreases and people lose weight as their disease progresses. This loss of appetite, known as anorexia,[7] appears when symptoms that affect the dying person's ability to eat (e.g., a sore mouth, difficulty swallowing, difficulty breathing) or symptoms that affect their interest in eating (e.g., pain, nausea, vomiting, constipation, depression, fatigue) occur. Anorexia is one contributor to the weight loss dying people experience.

Anorexia and Cachexia

People also lose weight as their disease progresses. A major contributor to weight loss is cachexia, wherein a person loses weight regardless of their intake. Considerable muscle tissue is lost when cachexia occurs, giving rise to the dramatic "wasted" appearance of dying people.

These two symptoms, anorexia and cachexia, can be very difficult for the person and family. PSWs can support the person and family by helping them understand the symptoms and adapt to the person's changing needs.

> **Food**
>
> Food is usually more than just fuel for the body.
>
> Food can communicate care, love, and concern.
>
> Food can nourish, strengthen, and support.
>
> Food is used to celebrate.
>
> Food is shared at times of mourning.

Decreased appetite and weight loss are difficult for family to witness

> Decreased intake and weight loss are two of the most common symptoms in the dying. These are also the most difficult symptoms for family and loved ones to witness.

---

7 In this text, anorexia is discussed only as it relates to caring for the dying.

Gathering Information

Observing

When a person has anorexia or cachexia you might observe the person:
- Has small and consistent decreases in eating
- Snacks rather than eating a full meal
- Chooses to miss meals
- Make comments such as "I'm not hungry now" at times when they previously enjoyed eating, states "The food is tasteless," "This drink doesn't taste good," or "Everything tastes the same"
- Looses weight involuntarily
- Has difficulty swallowing some or all of foods

Asking questions

To determine what these changes mean to the person, you can ask the person questions such as these:

I've noticed that your appetite seems different. Can you tell me about that?

Is there anything that makes you want to eat?

What makes it harder to eat?

What can I do to help?

Comfort Measures

Preventive

As the PSW, you can help the person and their family understand that decreases in appetite and weight loss are common changes as disease progresses. You can encourage the person and family to think of ways they can have quality time together that do not require the person to eat. Try to avoid doing painful procedures at mealtimes.

With the person and family, brainstorm ideas for spending time together without eating

In the moment

When the person's appetite starts to diminish, explore with the person their goals for intake. If the person wants to increase their intake, you might try the following:
- Make a list of the person's favourite foods and drinks, and use this information to help create the most desirable food options.
- Offer nutritious shakes and smoothies.
- Encourage the person and their family to meet with a dietitian to talk about nutrition and how to make good food choices when anorexia and cachexia are present. Alternatively, help the health care team provide nutritional information for the person and family to read.

What are the person's goals for intake?

It is important to respect the person's decisions about what they want to eat and how much to eat. Forcing a dying person to eat too much food can cause discomfort, bloating, nausea, and vomiting. As the person's intake decreases and the person is not interested in eating,

- Decrease portion sizes, providing very small meals more frequently
- Offer a comfort measure instead

Later in their disease process

As the person declines, these are some things to keep in mind:

- Continue to offer the person's preferred foods, checking frequently to see if their preferences have changed.
- Try to help the person see eating as something they choose to do, rather than as an obligation to please other people.
- For a person whose appetite is small, present food in easily managed portions, as in these examples:
  - Three grapes cut in half and two raspberries in a small bowl is a manageable amount, but a full cereal bowl of fruit is an unmanageably large portion.
  - One-eighth of a hardboiled egg and five very thin slices of cucumber on a small plate can be appetizing, but a full dinner plate of scrambled eggs is unmanageable.
- Depending on the person's energy level, vary the places for eating (e.g., in bed, by the bed, in the dining area, out on the sun deck).
- Suggest that the person have a quiet time or rest before eating so that they have the energy to eat.
- Position pillows to raise the person's head or maximize their comfort when eating.
- Sit and be with the person at times other than mealtimes, when food is not an intrusion.

As the person's body changes, you can help in these ways:

- Listen to the person's concerns about changes in their body image. (It is difficult to look in the mirror and not recognize the stranger looking back at you!)
- Record and report their concerns regarding appetite, weight loss, or intake to the nurse, social worker, dietitian, or other member of the health care team.

Ill-fitting dentures, mouth sores, and other problems in the mouth may cause the person discomfort and affect intake. You can help in these ways:

- Observe the person for any signs of discomfort.
- Encourage the person to report any discomfort.
- Maintain good mouth care.

For the family

It can be very upsetting for the family to witness the changes in their loved one as their intake decreases and their body becomes thinner. You can support the person and family by

- Listening to the family's concerns about their loved one's decreased intake and weight loss
- Witnessing the family's suffering and empathizing with their difficulty in seeing these changes in their loved one. You might say, for example,

    I can see it is difficult for you to watch your mom becoming thinner and eating so little.

- Recording and reporting the family's concerns to the health care team
- Helping the family obtain and understand accurate information about anorexia and cachexia, You can also encourage the family to talk about these aspects:
  - How the need for nourishment changes across a lifespan

    It is interesting how each person in the family has different needs for food.

  - The meaning of food and meals in their family, personally and culturally

    It must be hard not to bring him food when you have fed him and nourished him for years.

  - Different ways that a family can nurture

    What other things did you do for him that expressed love and care? Did you read to him, give him massages, play music for him, or tell him stories that remind him of his value and legacy?

Reminding the family about the following will also be helpful:

- The importance of sharing the social atmosphere of mealtimes with the person (e.g., having a small picnic on their bed together)
- Using strategies that the family has used in the past to nurture the person now
- That their loved one "is not dying because she is not eating; she is not eating because she is dying"

Good communication, education sessions to share information about expected changes, a consistent understanding and approach on the part of all team members, and opportunities to reflect on cultural and personal beliefs about food and what it means to support a loved one when they are not well may all help decrease stress when these changes are experienced.

Listen and empathize with the family

Help the family to nurture in ways that do not include food

> **Profound Truths of Nutrition**
>
> What a dying person can eat and drink decreases over time.
>
> Eventually, their eating and drinking will decrease to nothing.
>
> Stopping eating and drinking is natural in the dying process.
>
> What is nutritionally right at one stage may be very wrong at another.
>
> Pushing food on a person with advanced disease often worsens other symptoms.
>
> Food can cause more discomfort than pleasure.
>
> What a person likes is more important than what is "right" or "of value."
>
> What works is not necessarily what one likes or what is right.
>
> The atmosphere around eating is more important that what is ingested.

Medications and Treatments

Unfortunately, there are no medications or specific care strategies for treating or preventing anorexia or cachexia. Therefore, all treatments will be supportive only.

A few medications stimulate the appetite but are effective only if the person is able to digest food. A combination of medications may help the person gain weight in the short term. No medications reverse cachexia, increase energy over the long term, or prolong life.

More about Anorexia and Cachexia

Common questions about decreased appetite and involuntary weight loss

What is anorexia cachexia syndrome?

Decreased intake and involuntary weight loss can occur together or independently. When a person has both, their condition is termed "anorexia cachexia syndrome."

Research has shown that nutrition supplements in later stages of life do not prolong it and may not improve quality of life. Weight loss relates less to what the person eats or does not eat and more to what is *happening* inside their body.

What causes cachexia and anorexia?

When a person is very ill, their body's immune system triggers an inflammatory response. Current research indicates that the inflammatory response causes weight loss and decreases the appetite. It is important to note that weight loss occurs regardless of how much a person eats.

What causes weight loss?

The weight loss is partly the result of a poor appetite and decreased intake. When cachexia occurs, the inflammatory response consumes nutrients faster than they would normally be consumed. The body ends up using its own muscles to meet its nutrient needs, which results in weight loss.

Is cachexia the same as starvation?

Cachexia is different from starvation. When a person is starving, their body processes slow down to conserve nutrients, burning fat before muscle tissue for energy. With cachexia, the body processes speed up in response to the inflammation, consuming more energy than normal. In contrast to what happens in starvation, with cachexia the body burns muscle tissue for energy before fat tissue. This loss of muscle tissue greatly changes the appearance of the person, giving rise to the wasted look of cachexia.

Is she dying because she is not eating?

No. She is not eating because she is dying.

Is the dying person uncomfortable because they are not eating?

A dying person does not experience hunger in the same way that a healthy person does. Therefore, decreased intake in a dying person does not give rise to feelings of hunger. A dry mouth or other types of problems in the mouth cause discomfort, so regular mouth care will be helpful for a person with anorexia and cachexia.

How can you support and care for the person?

You can provide nurturing care in the form of skin care, massage, and mouth care. You can explore how to simply "be with" the person, providing companionship, for example, by reading to or telling the person stories. Ask the family how they would like to help.

Are there any treatments or medications that would help?

Medications can stimulate the appetite. Because there are many causes of anorexia and cachexia, the person may need a combination of medications. Current medications such as steroids do not increase weight over the long term, nor do they build muscle mass or prolong life.

Dehydration

The family called me into the room and told me, "Mom isn't drinking any water. Her mouth is dry. She is sleeping all the time. She does not wake up when we talk to her. Does she need some water? Is she comfortable?

Dehydration affects functioning of the:
- brain
- kidneys
- bowels
- bladder
- skin

Dehydration occurs when the fluid level in a person's body is less than that necessary to maintain normal body functions. Decreased fluid levels can affect kidney, liver, bowel, bladder, skin, and brain functions.

Gathering Information

Observing

When a person is dehydrated, their liquid intake is less than their liquid output. Symptoms that increase liquid output (e.g., vomiting, diarrhea) or that decrease liquid intake (e.g., nausea, bowel obstructions, decreased intake in the last days and hours) can cause a state of dehydration.

A dehydrated person may be uncomfortable due to the causes of the dehydration (e.g., nausea, vomiting, diarrhea) or the effects of the dehydration (e.g., mouth dryness, delirium). Dehydration may also contribute to comfort in the actively dying, by decreasing some symptoms (e.g., urinary output, nausea, vomiting, respiratory congestion). Therefore it is important to assess the dehydrated person's level of discomfort, as well as their goals for care.

Signs of dehydration

A person who is dehydrated may
- Feel and express thirst
- Develop a dry mouth, lips, and tongue
- Produce small amounts of dark urine
- Develop dry skin
- Lose skin firmness
- Become constipated
- Feel dizzy, drowsy, and tired
- Develop delirium

Asking questions

PSWs can gather information by asking symptom-appropriate questions like those in the List of Sample Questions.

Comfort Measures

Preventive

People at risk for dehydration are those who are losing more fluids than they are taking in. Therefore, you can help prevent dehydration by encouraging increased fluid intake and decreased fluid output in people at risk. If the person is vomiting, work with the health care team to decrease the person's nausea as quickly as possible. Use these strategies to minimize the risk of dehydration:

- Make sure the person's favourite drinks are within reach (e.g., on the bedside table) to encourage frequent drinking. If necessary, remind the person to drink by offering sips regularly.
- Encourage the person to avoid dehydrating liquids, such as coffee, black or green tea, and alcohol.
- Take measures to minimize dryness in the mouth, lips, and tongue and so prevent discomfort in the mouth.

Offer fluids when appropriate

Doing the following may help prevent dehydration in people who have difficulty swallowing:

- Offer liquids in thickened form (e.g., thickened soups).
- Offer clear fluids in solid form (e.g., flavoured gelatin, Popsicles).

In the moment

You can help a person who is dehydrated in these ways:

- Continue with preventive measures for dehydration.
- Continue to provide good mouth care.
- Instill eye drops if the person's eyes become dry.
- Reposition the person often to prevent sores caused by dehydration and skin breakdown.
- Massage pressure areas of the skin gently, avoiding areas that are reddened or white.

For the family

The person or their family may be concerned that dehydration is causing discomfort. You can encourage them to talk with the nurse and/or physician about their concerns in order to learn what options are available for managing the effects of dehydration.

In your practice, you can invite family members to participate in providing comfort to the dehydrated person and show them ways to do so (e.g., offer sips of fluids if appropriate, help provide good mouth care).

Encourage the family to share their concerns about decreased intake with the nurse, physician or dietitian

Refer to Chapter 6 for ways to support the family when their loved one is near death.

Medications and Treatments

Rehydrating a person who is dehydrated has advantages and disadvantages. The decision to rehydrate depends on the person's goals of care, the progress of their disease, and their comfort goals.

The cause of dehydration and the goals of care will help determine appropriate treatment

For example: A woman is dehydrated and has dry mouth, lips and tongue following vomiting associated with chemotherapy. She chose to receive chemotherapy to reduce tumour size and decrease pain. She is accepting of interventions to improve comfort. Artificial hydration would probably help her feel more comfortable and would probably be appropriate for this person at this time. Fluids can be given by intravenous route or hypodermoclysis.

A few months later this same woman is actively dying. She cannot swallow fluids and her mouth, tongue and lips are dry. She does not want any further invasive procedures. Excellent oral care on a regular basis improves her comfort. Based on her wishes, both she and family refuse artificial hydration.

> **Recent research found there was no difference in outcome between dying people who received one litre of fluid a day and those who did not.**[8]

The decision to rehydrate a person can be difficult and must be approached uniquely for each person. When the family has to make this decision, it can also be important for them to know they explored all options to ensure their loved one's comfort. In these cases, a 24-hour period of rehydration may be tried. The family will see how their loved one responds to the treatment, know they explored all options, and then can reconsider their decision about rehydration.

Team communication, education, and support of informed decision making will make it easier for the person and family dealing with dehydration.

More about Rehydration

Hypodermoclysis

Dehydration can be treated by rehydrating the person, either through intravenous (IV) fluids or by a less invasive procedure known as hypodermoclysis. In hypodermoclysis, fluids from an IV bag enter the fatty tissue under the skin through a needle. This fluid is absorbed slowly into the circulatory system and distributed throughout the body. Fatty open areas, such as the abdomen, thigh, upper back, or arm, are used for hypodermoclysis; however, the location of the needle that delivers the fluid is determined by the person's comfort. This subcutaneous route, which is easier to set up and less invasive than the IV route, may be preferred.

---

8   E. Bruera et al., "Parenteral Hydration in Patients with Advanced Cancer: A Multicenter, Double-Blind, Placebo-Controlled Randomized Trial," *Journal of Clinical Oncology* 31, no. 1 (2013): 111–118.

Delirium

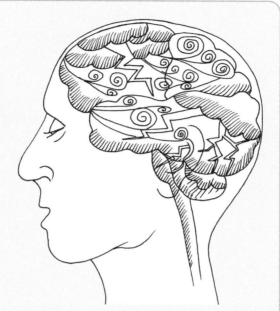

In order for me (the brain) to work, the rest of my body parts and organs have to work! If they don't do their job, then I can't do mine! If the body does not work well, then I get confused: I can't find the right words, pay attention, make clear decisions, remember things, or sort out what is past, present, or future! Sometimes I hallucinate and often I misunderstand. And worst of all, no one seems to understand me. Sometimes I am sleepy when I am supposed to be awake, and other times I am awake when everyone else is trying to sleep. Sometimes I get agitated and upset, and other times I am just sleepy and wonder what the fuss is all around me. Sometimes I see things that no one else sees. Sometimes the things I see make sense (like the time I mistook the nurse for my daughter, or the time I thought the bells were the fire alarm when my house burned down), but other times, the images that I see are scary, and I am scared.

I understand that what I experience is called "delirium." When I am in the midst of this delirium, I can't always answer questions about it, but then, a little while later, I might be clear enough to tell you my memories. In fact, we might even be able to find themes and reasons for the delirium.

When I ask the nurse why delirium occurs, I am told a whole list of things. But one thing that no one mentions is dying. Do you know, if you look at most of the causes of delirium, most occur naturally in the dying process? And in addition to the things within my body that cause delirium, medications are a really common cause of it, and my body and I, we often need some of these medications that cause delirium in order to manage common symptoms of dying. So as I see it, dying causes delirium.

Let me tell you why …

My body and I, we are connected. My body is sick right now. As the disease progresses through my body, my desire for food and my ability to swallow and digest food decrease. My organs, including my kidneys, liver, and heart, are not functioning well. My metabolism is changing. I am low on water and oxygen, and my electrolytes are out of balance.

The toxins are building up. My immune system is weak. I get more infections—urinary tract infections and pneumonia are my constant companions. In order to do their job well, the antibiotics need a healthy immune system, so in my body they can't do their job well. I expect that at some point the antibiotics will stop working altogether!

Oh, and my bladder and bowels aren't working well, and with the side effects of medications, the bowels gets constipated. Let me tell you, when the bowel is constipated, I can't see straight!

The long and short of it is, you can look at the list of all the different things that cause delirium, but dying … well, dying is the "perfect storm" for delirium.

Stanley was unable to recognize family visitors yesterday. Last night he could not sleep and was up and down all night long. He did not know what he wanted, but he wanted something. This morning he got up and put his shaving kit into the freezer and pulled out pages from his crossword book to clean the counter. When I arrived, we talked and he kept falling asleep. Now he won't wake up. I was supposed to give him a bath today. I am thinking that I will just give him a bed bath.

Delirium[9] is a physical state in which the brain cannot send and receive information correctly. The person with delirium is confused, easily distracted, and unable to focus on tasks or conversations. Their consciousness may be altered, and they may alternately be alert, agitated, or drowsy. The person may hallucinate, incorrectly interpret information (e.g., may not know where they are or why), and may be unable to communicate their thoughts or needs effectively. The confusion can cause feelings of fear and paranoia. The state of delirium can be reversible or irreversible, lasting a few hours or days, occurring repeatedly as disease progresses, or indicating imminent death.

---

9 In this text, "near-death awareness"—a state in which a dying person sees loved ones who have previously died—is not considered to be delirium. Near-death (or "pre-death") awareness is discussed in Chapter 6.

Gathering Information

Observing

Delirium refers to *sudden*[10] changes in a person's mental processes of attention, memory, producing and understanding language, learning, reasoning, problem solving, and decision making. You should suspect delirium in a person who suddenly displays symptoms such as the following:

- Difficulty focusing on a task or conversation
- Difficulty communicating (e.g., forming sentences or understanding people)
- Difficulty reasoning through a problem (e.g., finding their shoes)
- Difficulty making simple decisions (e.g., deciding what they would like for breakfast)
- Difficulty remembering events from earlier in the day or the previous day
- Fear or paranoia (e.g., saying things such as "I'm afraid" or "That nurse is really mean to me")
- A disturbed sleep–wake cycle (e.g., is up in the middle of the night wandering around, but then can't stay awake during the day)

When talking with family members, you may hear them express their fatigue:

We just can't keep up because he is getting into everything and he doesn't make sense.

Asking questions

It may be difficult to obtain information from a person with delirium, so you will probably need to direct your questions to the family, or consider your own observations of the person. You can use the following questions, adapted from questions in the Confusion Assessment Method,[11] to explore sudden changes in the person.

1. Mental processing
- When did you first notice the change?
- Before this change, when was the last time you observed that the person's mentation was normal?
- Does the person's lack of concentration vary during the day?

2. Level of attention
- Is the person more easily distracted than previously?
- Does the person have difficulty following what is being said or done?

---

10 In terms of delirium, the word "sudden" is used to describe a change that happens quickly, occurring over one hour or a day. In comparison, changes due to dementia occur over months and years.

11 The Confusion Assessment Method is a standardized tool used to identify delirium quickly.

3. Speech and language skills
- Does the person's speech sound jumbled, like a word salad?
- Is the person's speech a random unpredictable flow of conversation, switching from one subject to another?
- Does the person understand you when you talk with them?

4. Level of consciousness
- Is the person lethargic or difficult to wake?
- Is the person acutely alert or vigilant?
- Does the person seem to be highly aroused or agitated?
- Is the person unable to settle or sleep?

Differences between Delirium and Dementia

Delirium and dementia look different

Distinguishing between delirium and dementia can be difficult because people with these conditions may behave in similar ways. Knowing the person's history will help the health care team determine whether the person has a delirium or dementia. Comparing delirium to dementia uncovers the following differences, as well as one similarity:

What it is: Delirium is a change in a person's mental abilities, whereas dementia is a brain disease.

Sudden onset: Delirium develops suddenly over hours or a day, whereas dementia develops gradually and shows slow, steady changes over months and years.

Reversibility: Changes caused by delirium may be reversible. Dementia is not reversible.

Hallucinations: A person with delirium may experience hallucinations. This does not usually happen with dementia (except with Lewy Body type dementia).

Causes: Delirium is caused by changes in the body (e.g., fever, infection, dehydration, decreased kidney/liver function, electrolyte imbalances) that affect how the brain is able to work. Dementia is caused by permanent changes in the brain tissues (e.g., formation of plaques in the case of Alzheimer's disease).

Common symptoms: Anxiety, fear, and paranoia are symptoms of both delirium and dementia.

Comfort Measures

You can support and comfort a person with delirium by providing them with familiar items and care. Personal things, photos, and stories from their past can provide a sense of security and safety. Delirium may bring up incidents from a person's life that might increase misunderstandings, anxiety, and stress. The family may have insight into these incidents that will help you comfort the person during a period of delirium. People who have experienced violent trauma in their past quite often revisit the experience when in a delirium. Being aware of the person's history of trauma will help you provide comfort during the person's delirium.

Familiar objects may comfort a person with delirium

Preventive

Many of the physical changes of dying (e.g., infections, dehydration, medication side effects, constipation, electrolyte imbalances) can cause delirium. You can help minimize a person's chance of developing severe delirium in the following ways:

Common changes with dying also cause delirium

- Be alert for signs of delirium. Report the delirium as soon as possible. Do not wait for the delirium to escalate before reporting it.
- Provide a quiet, familiar, safe environment with adequate lighting.
- Maintain the person's daily routines as much as possible.
- Support consistent staffing to minimize confusion for the person.
- Record and report the person's history of delirium, as well as their history of traumatic themes that emerge in dreams.
- If the person is receiving opioids and is able to swallow, offer liquids to help their body get rid of the byproducts of the medication.

During delirium

During delirium, the person is not able to direct their own care, cannot manage their own safety, and may be in an altered state. This section describes what you will need to provide in caring for a person experiencing delirium.

Personal safety
It is important to ensure that the person in your care is safe:

- Make sure that the person does not have access to objects with which they could harm themselves or others (e.g., scissors, knives, sharp tools, medications).
- If the person tries to get out of bed on their own, keep the side rails of the bed down and lower the bed. If necessary, place a mattress on the floor beside the bed in case the person falls.
- Report immediately if a delirious person shows signs that they will cause themselves or others physical harm. Avoid using physical restraints that may increase a person's physical aggression.

Emotional security
A person who is experiencing an altered reality due to delirium may benefit from the emotional support provided by the presence of a friend or family member. Known as companioning, this can reduce anxiety and help the person orient to

reality. Family may be able to companion, but they might find the person's confusion very difficult to witness and may not want to sit for long periods with someone whose condition is not settling.

Appropriate communications

Delirium affects the person's ability to speak and to understand language. Supporting a person with delirium requires that you speak in simple, clear, short sentences. Be patient when speaking, ask one question at a time, and wait for an answer before proceeding. For example, ask

Are you thirsty?

Would you like a blanket?

instead of

Can I get you a drink? A meal? Are you hungry? How about a blanket—are you warm enough? That's what I am here for.

Orientation to reality

Explore the dying person's reality to determine what they are experiencing. If possible, orient them to reality. These are some questions you might ask the person:

What do you see? What do you hear?

Are you worried about something?

Tell me how this is for you.

Reassurance

Delirium will make it difficult for the person to remember and understand what is happening. You can help them through the difficulties of delirium by reminding them frequently that they are not alone:

I am here with you. I will make sure you are safe.

Support during hallucinations

Hallucinations can terrify a person. You will need to work to understand what they are experiencing and then reassure them that you are there to help.

I don't see the spiders, but I know that you see them and I am here to help make them go away.

Spiritual support

A religious person may interpret visions due to delirium as demonic or evil, which could be frightening in light of their religious beliefs. In such cases, seek the support of a spiritual advisor who would be comforting for the person.

During delirium, remember:
- safety
- emotional security
- communication
- orientation
- reassurance
- support
- relaxation

Relaxation

Helping a person with delirium to relax can be supportive and provide a break for the family. Offering these comfort measures may help the person relax:

- Warmed blankets
- Soft items (e.g., stuffed toy animal, soft fleece blanket)
- Reiki, massage, or Healing Touch support
- Favourite music
- Aromatherapy

When the delirium has stopped

Sometimes people remember their experience of being confused, others do not remember. If the person expresses concerns you may want to explain that sometimes people experience delirium, and that they are not "going crazy". You may hear the person talk about issues such as these:

People may need reassurance after experiencing delirium

- Their delirium

  I was terrified. I thought the house was burning down.

- Fears and embarrassment

  I apologize, I think I was confused and really upset earlier today.

- Concerns about being a burden
- Feeling vulnerable
- A theme of their delirium and how it relates to their life, dying, and disease
- Their concerns about the difference between delirium and pre-death awareness.

For the family

A loved one's delirium can be frightening for family members to witness, and the family may need as much support as the dying person. You can help the family by

- Listening to their concerns and reporting these to the nurse
- Providing reassurance that the loved one's delirium does not mean they are crazy
- Providing a space for the family to nap and regain their strength during the delirium or after the person settles
- Providing warm blankets or other comfort items

The family may want to talk with the nurse about themes that came forward in the delirium. They may also have questions for the nurse or health care team about the differences between delirium and pre-death awareness.

Medications and Treatments

Medications can help manage symptoms of delirium, such as paranoia, hallucinations, and insomnia. The person's goal of care will direct the physician, health care team, and family when they make decisions about medications. Consider the care plans in these two scenarios:

My dad just wants to be comfortable. He does not want any further tests or treatments.

Dad was clear this morning and he wants to live for the anniversary party this weekend. I think it is important to him for this delirium to be investigated and treated if possible.

Sample Report

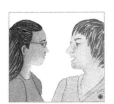 66 *I am calling about Mr. Preet. PPS 40%. Tonight his daughter Sushila and I transferred him to bed. He became confused. He demanded to have his socks removed and did not get into bed until Sushila removed two imaginary socks from his feet. Seeing him confused made me reflect on how he was earlier today. This afternoon he was very distracted by a conversation in the next room. He could not focus on the person visiting him. He also got his words mixed up. This is a change for him. He is normally totally clear. He has been eating only tiny amounts in the past few days. He is weaker with transfers. Can you see him?* 99

Medications can help to manage symptoms associated with delirium, but are not able to reverse the delirium.

Difficult Breathing

I walked into her room. She was hunched over at the side of the bed and gasping for air. I pulled up the over-bed table and helped her sit up and lean with her arms on the table for support. I opened the window, turned the fan on, and pushed the commode out of her room. She looked frightened and pale. She nodded as though to greet me.

I called for the nurse: "Mina is gasping and struggling to breathe. Please come now."

I knelt in front of her, took her hand in mine, looked her in the eyes, and said, "I will stay with you. The nurse is coming and she will get you some medication to help you breathe more comfortably."

I started breathing to match her breaths. Then slowly I coached her to breathe with me, and she started to breathe more slowly. The nurse arrived, assessed her, and provided the medication as ordered.

Difficult breathing, also called dyspnea, is the uncomfortable sensation of struggling to breathe, the feeling of being unable get enough air. Difficult breathing is a common symptom and can be a very distressing one for the dying person and their family. Therefore, it is important for PSWs to be alert for symptoms that indicate difficult breathing.

Difficult breathing = dyspnea

Gathering Information

It is not always possible to know by looking at a person that they are having difficulty breathing. A person with dyspnea, also known as shortness of breath, may breathe faster than normal, they may look like they are working hard to breathe, or they may look like they are breathing normally. A person working hard to breathe will usually answer yes when asked if they are feeling short of breath. If the person is not asked, however, they may not report their difficulty with breathing until the symptom is quite severe.

Observing

Be alert to behaviours, such as those below, that indicate the person is experiencing difficult breathing:

1. Shortness of breath
A person with difficult breathing may
  - Pause to breathe halfway through a sentence or during any activity
  - Gasp for air when moving or at rest
  - Open their mouth wide to get more air
  - Purse their lips when breathing

Consider difficult breathing when you observe these behaviours

- Use neck, shoulder, and back accessory muscles to help breathe
- Refuse to participate in activities so as to avoid or reduce breathlessness

2. Changes in respiratory patterns, sounds, and rates
A person with difficult breathing may
- Be congested and have moist, wheezy, or raspy breath sounds
- Have a cough accompanied by sounds of dryness or congestion
- Breathe with shallow, quick breaths

3. Managing difficulty breathing on their own
A person trying to manage difficult breathing on their own may
- Move, change position, and shift around (e.g., bend over with elbows on knees to catch their breath) to increase their lung capacity
- Sleep upright in a recliner
- Feel agitated and restless
- Express surprise and fright

  > *I couldn't breathe. I thought I was dying.*

- Talk about fatigue and lack of energy

  > *I have no energy today.*

  > *I am so tired.*

  > *I don't think I can get up today.*

4. Comments by the family
Family members may make comments about the person's state, such as these:

> *My husband is so weak, he can hardly get out of bed.*

> *My mom is so tired, she doesn't get up.*

Asking questions

At a time when the person is not in distress, you can invite the person to tell you about their difficult breathing by asking questions such as these:
- When did your difficult breathing start?
- How do you feel when you have difficult breathing?
- Can you rate your difficult breathing on a scale?
  - 0 to 10 (0 = no symptom and 10 = the worst imaginable)
  - Small, medium, large
  - Mild, moderate, severe
- What makes it easier to breathe?
- What makes it harder to breathe?
- What can I do to help you when you have difficult breathing?

Ask questions when the person *is not* experiencing difficulty breathing

You may not need to ask these questions if the nurse or other members of the health care team are available and able to assess. If the nurse is not available, then you may need to gather information that will help the team decide how best to respond.

Comfort Measures

Preventive

People experience difficult breathing for many different reasons. Asking questions and observing the person's responses to items in their environment will help you determine triggers that may cause difficulty breathing. Observe for things that help settle the person's difficult breathing to help avoid future episodes.

You can help a person manage difficult breathing by
- Investigating triggers that lead to difficult breathing in the person
- Planning ways to avoid these triggers as much as possible
- Ensuring that unnecessary airway irritants (e.g., perfumes, powders, sprays) are not used around the person

Be alert for triggers of difficult breathing

When physical activity causes or worsens difficult breathing, people may benefit by
- Pacing their activities, including those of daily living, to avoid triggering difficulty breathing
- Moving slowly during and between activities
- Resting and recovering between activities
- Avoiding hurrying or introducing any sense of urgency
- Stopping to rest and pause to breathe between one action and the next in a sequence
- Using physical supports for their arms (e.g., resting their elbows on a physical support when using their arms to eat, shave, or brush their teeth)
- Limiting all or some visitors, or limiting the length of visits as necessary

In the moment

A person experiencing difficult breathing may be anxious, fearful, and/or confused. You can support them by remaining calm and staying with them while calling for the nurse. These are some strategies that may help a person experiencing difficult breathing:

Remain calm and stay with the person experiencing difficulty breathing

- Provide air flow around the person by opening windows and curtains or using a table fan.
- Coach the person to breathe slowly, using a calming low voice. It may help some people to focus on you and for you to coach them in their breathing, as in these examples:

> *Look into my eyes and breathe with me.* (Breathe slowly and audibly slow your breathing as you coach the person.)

After a few slower breaths, reassure the person:

> *Good, keep breathing with me … your breathing is slowing down … you are doing fine … you are doing a good job of breathing slowly … just breathe … slowly and steadily … The oxygen is getting to your body, you are doing well.*

Continue in this manner if it is helpful until the person is more comfortable.

Explore positions that may help relieve difficult breathing

- Position the person to increase their lung volume and hopefully decrease their feeling of breathlessness. This may include returning a recliner chair back to the upright position, elevating the head of the bed, helping the person sit forward with their upper body and arms supported by pillows or the over-bed table, and suggesting that they lie on one side or the other, depending on their own preference.

For the family

Support family by listening and validating their concerns

The family could be upset by watching a loved one have difficulty with breathing. Share information about triggers that may cause difficult breathing in the person, and invite the family to participate in helping the person avoid or manage these triggers. Listen to the family's questions and fears, and refer the family to the nurse for more information.

Medication and Treatment

Medications may be helpful in decreasing those conditions that cause difficult breathing, or in decreasing the person's sensation of breathlessness. The doctor may order medications to reduce inflammation, dry up lung secretions, or lower a person's anxiety.

Opioids work by decreasing the feeling of breathlessness and thereby improve the person's quality of life. Using opioids can help a person continue in their favourite activities for a longer time. For people with advancing illness who are experiencing shortness of breath, opioids can be used early in the disease process, in addition to medications to treat the underlying causes. Opioids do not need to be reserved for the last days or weeks of a person's life.

Oxygen treatment

Oxygen therapy may not help decrease difficult breathing

People may believe that oxygen will fix breathing difficulties. Generally, providing more oxygen helps only when blood oxygen levels are low. Unfortunately, many people who commonly experience difficult breathing have normal or slightly low blood oxygen levels. Although they feel breathless and their body is working hard to breathe, they may be able to keep blood oxygen levels high enough such that providing more oxygen wouldn't help. In these instances, air movement on the person's face can be quite helpful. The health care team will need to assess the person and the cause of their difficult breathing to determine whether providing oxygen would help them.

Keep in mind the flammability and explosive nature of oxygen. When providing a person with oxygen, avoid using petroleum-based products or wool blankets and ensure that no one smokes nearby.

Depending on the person's goals of care and the progression of disease, asking a respiratory therapist or a physiotherapist for advice could be helpful.

Sample Record

••• PPS 40%. I went into Mina's room, and she was struggling to breathe, gasping for air. I called the nurse. Assisted to reposition Mina up, arms up over the over-bed table, opened window, turned on the fan, removed the commode, coached her to breathe with me. Nurse arrived, administered. Half an hour later Mina reported breathing was comfortable and is resting while sitting up in the recliner. •••

Sample Report

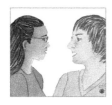

66 Thanks for coming to see Mina. I just went back to check on her, and she is more relaxed, sitting up in her recliner, and says that her breathing is comfortable. 99

I was interested in the idea of coaching someone to breathe when they are struggling to breathe comfortably. So, one day I tried it.

I work with a man who is 94 and has congestive heart failure. When he is anxious or stressed, his breathing becomes rapid and shallow. When he gets his morning care, he gets short of breath. One day I tried to coach him. I started breathing with him, at the same pace, quick and shallow. Then I slowly started breathing deeper and slower. He followed me and within 30 to 40 seconds he was breathing more comfortably. This was easy, it was personal, and it was a great comfort to him, to his wife who was watching, and to me—I had something to do that was supportive. My co-workers and I will continue to use this.

—Jackie McDonald

Fatigue

Energy is such a funny thing—it feels as if it just drains right out of me. It is like I have just a tablespoon of energy, and when it is gone, instead of filling up quickly, it might take a day resting to recover. It is like the tap refuelling me only refills a drop at a time.
—Yetta Lees

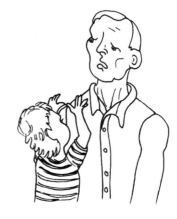

Fatigue feels different for everyone. Healthy people feel fatigued after using energy (e.g., after exercise, after a day at work, at the end of an exam). When a person has a progressive life-threatening illness, they may feel fatigued without having consciously used any energy. Fatigue is often an early sign of illness and usually becomes more obvious as disease progresses. Disease alone can cause fatigue, or fatigue may result from medication, stress, decreased intake, weight loss, treatments, sleep disturbances, depression, fears, anxiety, and pain.

Fatigue without exertion can be an early sign of illness

Gathering Information

Observing

Fatigue without prior exertion can be an early sign of disease. A PSW would suspect fatigue if the person
- Couldn't complete their activities of daily living and other usual tasks
- Slept or rested for more time than usual but arose without feeling refreshed or energized
- Said things like "I am still so tired" or "I slept all day and I could sleep all night"
- Started a task but was not able to complete it
- Felt distressed after engaging in even with limited activities
- Withdrew from or lost interest in activities
- Refused to see visitors

Asking questions

If you observe fatigue in the person you are caring for, you can adapt the questions in the List of Sample Questions to create your own questions to use in exploring what you have observed, determine whether the person is fatigued, and individualize comfort measures for fatigue.

Comfort Measures

Although fatigue can be very distressing for the dying person, PSWs may overlook it while managing more obvious symptoms such as pain, nausea, and delirium. You can support a person by listening to them and their family talk about fatigue and discussing it with them. Bearing witness to their frustration and limitations will acknowledge the reality of the fatigue.

Be mindful of the person's energy when providing care. When the person is fatigued, you may want to be quiet, gentle, and positive rather than energetic and enthusiastic in your conversation.

Preventive

PSWs can support a fatigued person by helping them with their activities of daily living. You could open the conversation by saying,

> *I am here to help do the things that are of less interest to you so that you can use your energy for things that are most important to you.*

To help the person pace their plans for the day, you might say,

> *I notice that you have more energy in the morning and are tired and want to sleep in the afternoon. Do you want your family to visit you in the morning?*
>
> *Would you like to limit the number of visitors or limit the length of their visits?*

Early in the disease process, the physiotherapist may discuss the benefits of exercise as a way to increase energy. As disease progresses, exercise may add to exhaustion.

Preventing fatigue is supportive care

In the moment

When a person is fatigued, you might offer to
- Reschedule treatments and activities
- Provide the person with a meal in bed
- Offer a small snack rather than a full meal
- Suggest activities that are relaxing (e.g., listening to music, massage)

Being flexible in providing care can help a person maintain their limited energy

When nighttime sleep becomes disturbed, you can suggest options that could improve sleep, such as having a quiet time before bed, listening to music, and receiving therapeutic touch or a comforting visit by a loved one.

For the family

PSWs can help the family understand the changing energy levels of the dying person. It is helpful to work with family to plan appropriate activities and caregiving that will meet their needs and those of the fatigued person. Always listen to family members to understand their concerns, and acknowledge their fears about what fatigue might mean for the person. Report the family's concerns (e.g., fatigue is caused by medications) to the nurse.

Planning and
mindfulness will help
when managing fatigue

When appropriate, invite the family to help the person with activities of daily living. Look for opportunities to share information with the family about how to

- Help their loved one without "doing it all" for them
- Be open to adapting plans daily or hourly, depending on how the person is feeling
- Be mindful, when visiting the person, of their energy and needs
- Revise the care plan with the nurse as determined by the person's needs
- Ask the nurse for more information about fatigue

You can also help the family by reinforcing the following messages provided by the health care team:

- Drowsiness is a normal side effect when a person begins to take opioids or when the opioid dose increases. The person's drowsiness will fade after a few days.
- As death nears, it is normal and expected that people will become weaker and sleep more.

Medications and Treatments

The person benefits most when treatments remove the cause of fatigue (e.g., antibiotics to remove infection, blood transfusion to treat anemia). When it is not possible to remove the cause of fatigue, a short course of steroids can boost the person's energy. This option is most helpful when a person wants to participate in certain activities (e.g., daily activities, an event such as a wedding). When the person's fatigue is so great that they cannot get out of bed, steroid medications will no longer work and are discontinued.

Mouth Discomfort

Most of the people I care for have dementia. They can't tell me when something is wrong. They can't tell me that they have a sore mouth. So I listen like I am a detective. I observe really carefully, I "listen to behaviours." Then I try to figure out what could be wrong.

I remember one lady who was upset, but she couldn't tell me what was wrong. She hit me and resisted care. Finally I started singing with her, and she relaxed a bit, I sat next to her.

Then I thought, "I need to see her mouth. She has not been letting me give her mouth care for the last few days. Sure enough, her mouth was ugly with red patches and creamy white spots sloughing off. She had a thrush infection. That had to be the cause of the pain.

Mouth discomfort develops when the normal tissues of the oral cavity become dry, irritated, and/or infected. There are many causes of mouth discomfort (e.g., medication side effects, poorly fitting dentures, a weakened immune system); therefore, preventive mouth care is important. Because PSWs provide the majority of personal care, they will be the first to notice changes in a person's mouth or their behaviour that may signal mouth pain.

PSWs are likely to notice signs of mouth discomfort first

Gathering Information

Observing

Some people may tell you their mouth is sore, but most people manage their sore mouth by avoiding activities that cause mouth pain. PSWs need to watch for behaviours that may signal mouth pain. A person who suddenly does not want anything in their mouth (e.g., refuses food, drinks less than usual, doesn't want their teeth cleaned) may have a sore mouth. If talking causes pain, the person may stop talking or moan instead of using words. If you see these behaviours, look further for symptoms of mouth discomfort.

Decreased eating may indicate mouth discomfort

The person with mouth discomfort may have
- Visibly dry lips, gums, or tongue
- Swollen mucosa, lips, or tongue
- Fresh or dried blood in their mouth or on their lips
- A coloured discharge on their toothbrush after use
- An unpleasant smell in the mouth
- Colour changes with or without red or white sores in their mouth
- Difficulty swallowing

Asking questions

You can adapt the questions in the List of Sample Questions to create your own questions to use in exploring and developing an understanding of the person's mouth discomfort and to individualize comfort measures.

Comfort Measures

Providing mouth care regularly will help prevent mouth dryness and sores. The preventive mouth care strategies discussed below are useful for all people receiving supportive care and are especially important for those at high risk for developing thrush infections (e.g., during and after radiation or chemotherapy). Focus on hydrating and lubricating the mouth in people at risk for dry mouth, such as those with limited intake or in who are in their last days and hours.

Preventive

Good mouth care can prevent mouth discomfort

It is important to use these mouth care strategies:
- Provide mouth care before and after the person eats.
- Remove the person's dentures before providing mouth care.
- Brush gently or wipe the mucosa to remove plaque and debris.
- For people resisting mouth care, use creative strategies to complete the task (e.g., distract them with singing, talking, gently touching).
- If the person has a thrush infection, soak their dentures and toothbrushes in a vinegar or disinfectant solution to prevent spreading the infection.
- Use a soft toothbrush and, if necessary, a specialized toothpaste.

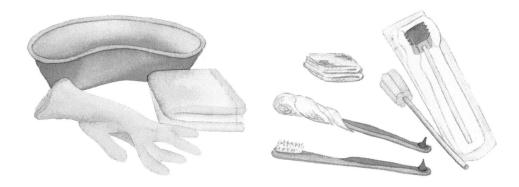

In the moment

Hydrate and lubricate to manage sore mouth

In addition to using the mouth care strategies listed above, if the person's mouth is dry, use these strategies to hydrate and lubricate:
- Offer water or other drinks frequently.
- Spray the inside of the person's mouth with cold water.
- Offer them ice cubes wrapped in a clean washcloth to moisten the mouth.
- Offer them slightly thawed Popsicles, pineapple chunks, sour candies, or chewing gum.

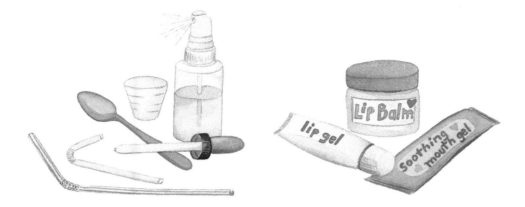

When a person cannot manage their own mouth care, you can use these strategies:

- Moisten their mouth mucosa gently using packaged or homemade mouth swabs.
- Offer these liquids to rinse their mouth:
  - Water
  - Salt water (1 teaspoon table salt mixed into 2 cups boiled and cooled water)
  - Alcohol-free germicidal mouthwash diluted to half strength with water
  - Brandy diluted with water to remove crusts and reduce breath odour
  - Club soda to loosen materials on mucosa and teeth
- Apply lubricant to the oral mucosa using a swab, after the mouth has been cleaned and rinsed.
- Apply lip balm after applying the lubricant (use water-based products if the person is receiving oxygen).
- Use a humidifier in the room to moisten the person's dry airways.

Individualize care

For the family

Invite the family to participate in mouth care as one way to support their loved one. Remind them to use gloves if the person has a thrush infection.

Medications and Treatments

Medications may be necessary for pain relief, to prevent or treat infections, and to encourage healing. Topical treatments may be "swish and swallow" or "swish and spit" depending on the medication. Report to the nurse when a person is not able to swallow or spit. Depending on your scope of practice, you may be directed to "paint" medication on with mouth swabs or to squirt medication onto the inner cheeks using a syringe.

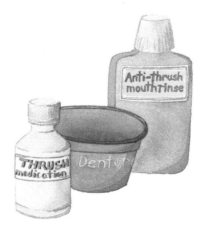

I need to be creative with this lady to get her comfortable. I set up towels, toothbrush, glass of water, and the rinse she is supposed to use for the thrush infection.

She loves singing, so I sing with her and walk her slowly into the bathroom. Using a singsong voice, I ask her if she would like to brush her teeth or rinse her mouth. Sometimes it takes several tries.

I try putting the toothbrush in her hand while singing or smiling, speaking softly to her. Then I gently lift the toothbrush to her mouth (keeping my fingers crossed she will work with me).

I always watch her body language. I stop when she gets defensive or agitated and switch the conversation to something she enjoys.

Sample Record

••• Brought resident into bathroom to do mouth care. PPS 30%. She refused to brush teeth but did rinse mouth with prescription mouth rinse. Mouth has red patches and creamy white spots still visible. No blood present in expelled rinse. No verbal expression of pain or facial expression of pain. Resident tolerated rinsing only if staff sang to her. No responsive behaviours present. Reported to nurse. Will continue to try to have resident brush teeth after meals and rinse her mouth as per orders. •••

Sample Report

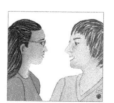

❝ Mrs. Z—I gave Mrs. Z mouth care. Red patches and creamy white spots still visible, there was no pain or blood, she was only able to rinse her mouth but did not allow me to brush her teeth. She enjoyed my singing while trying to do the mouth care. I charted the care and observations. ❞

Nausea and Vomiting

She was crying on the bed when I entered her room.

"I'm so tired of this nausea, I wish I could just die."

I sat with her and held her hand … It was all I could think of to help at that moment.

When she was less distressed, we talked of the things that make it worse and those things that might make it better. We made a few changes and then I phoned the nurse to report.

Nausea is a feeling of discomfort centred in a person's stomach and extending up their throat. Sometimes nausea creates the feeling there is a lump at the back of the throat. These feelings of discomfort can range from mild to severe. Nausea is often, but not always, accompanied by vomiting, that is, the contents of the stomach and digestive system moving in the reverse direction, coming up the esophagus and out through the mouth. These two symptoms can be very difficult for a person to tolerate, often as difficult as severe pain.

Working quickly to manage the causes and effects of nausea and vomiting or relieving the symptoms greatly improves a dying person's comfort. This can be difficult, however, because there are many causes (e.g., medication side effects, pain, stomach irritation, brain swelling, anxiety, odours). As PSWs provide most of the personal support for the person, your input is valuable when identifying the causes of nausea or vomiting. PSWs are also important in providing support for people experiencing nausea and vomiting.

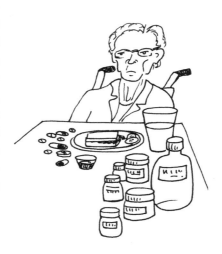

Responding quickly to nausea and vomiting can greatly improve the person's comfort

Gathering Information

Observing

People with nausea may not talk about mild nausea or say, "I feel nauseated." This means that the PSW needs to be aware of how people signal they are feeling nauseated. For example, a mildly nauseated person might say, "I don't feel good" or "My stomach is jumping" or "I have an upset tummy." When nausea increases, the person may tell you, "I think I am going to throw up" or "I'm going to be sick."

People describe nausea in different ways

Consider exploring whether a person is experiencing nausea if they
- Say "my stomach doesn't feel good" or "I have an upset stomach"
- Burp much more frequently than usual

- Begin taking deep breaths, possibly holding their breath for a short time, and placing pressure on their abdomen using their hands and arms
- Suddenly decrease their intake of or refuse food and drink
- Begin rocking or any type of repetitive continuous movement for no apparent reason.
- Make retching and gagging sounds

If the person vomits, observe and record the date and time they vomited and a description of what they vomited, including the amount, texture, and colour.

Asking questions

If you suspect a person is nauseated or if they have vomited, record and report
- The person's colouring, paleness, or pallor
- Their comments about feeling heartburn, stomach pain, or discomfort
- The date and description of the last bowel movement
- Any other symptoms, such as headache or anxiety

You can adapt the questions in the List of Sample Questions to create your own questions to use in exploring and developing an understanding of the person's nausea and vomiting. Adjust the comfort measures to meet the specific needs of the person.

Comfort Measures

Preventive

Understanding the cause of a person's nausea and vomiting can help prevent future episodes. As a PSW, you will be able to manage environmental causes of nausea and vomiting and help with personal care after vomiting.

Provide fresh air

When you suspect that the person you are caring for is experiencing nausea, taking the following actions will provide comfort:
- Removing from the room sources of unpleasant odours (e.g., commode, uneaten food)
- Ensuring that the flow of air in the room is sufficient to keep it smelling fresh and clean
- Using a bathroom fan to keep air moving

Preventive measures for vomiting include these:
- Providing regular mouth care, including rinsing the mouth after the person has vomited
- Supplying small meals that cater to the person's preferences and appetite on any given day
- Using pillows to help the person remain upright after eating if this position decreases nausea or vomiting

In the moment

When a person feels nauseated, you may help them feel better by

- Repositioning them to raise their head above the heart level, using pillows if necessary
- Providing fresh air by opening windows or using a fan

It is important to listen to the person's concerns, remembering that focusing on nausea can increase the feeling of nausea. Explore these options to help manage the person's symptoms:

- Ask if scents or perfumes are contributing to their symptoms.
- Ask whether visitors or quiet time would help.
- Offer distractions, for example, ask whether they would like to watch TV or listen to music.
- Offer gentle massage or other touch therapies if helpful.
- Connect with the care team to share information about managing nausea for this person.

Individualize measures for managing nausea by listening to the person

If the person is vomiting, in addition to initiating and continuing support for nausea as detailed above, you can also

- Provide privacy while the person is vomiting
- Offer mouth care after they have vomited
- Frequently offer small sips of fluids or ice chips to prevent dehydration
- Provide fresh sheets, towels, and sleepwear after the person has vomited

You will need to report to the nurse when the person stops vomiting and the nausea settles, and work with the team to adapt the care plan when the person wants to eat again. Once nausea and vomiting stop, the person may begin to take clear fluids and, if they are tolerated, can try full fluids and eventually progress to eating small meals.

For the family

If the person has specific preferences about who can be present when they are vomiting or being cleaned up after such episodes, you can help by communicating these preferences to the family. Explain that for some people vomiting can be embarrassing, as well as extremely uncomfortable. The family can help by gathering materials that will be needed if vomiting occurs (e.g., large bowls rather than small kidney-shaped basins, towels, washcloths, toothbrush, drinking glass). You might also consider doing the following if vomiting is expected:

- To make cleanup easier, pour a small amount of water into the bowl or bucket before the person vomits.
- Make non-see-through bags into which the person can vomit, by putting a plastic bag inside a small paper bag, because hiding the vomit can reduce their nausea. Once a bag has been used, you or the family can examine the contents and estimate the volume if there is concern about what is in the vomit.

Tips to manage nausea and clean up after vomiting

Medications and Treatments

As with pain, a combination of medications may be required to manage nausea and vomiting. Depending on the cause of the nausea or vomiting, the person may need to take the medication through until death. The dying person and their family may wonder why they have to keep taking the medication when they are no longer experiencing the symptoms. If the person or family talks about wanting to stop the medication when the symptom stops, suggest that they speak with the nurse or physician about this concern.

Sample Report

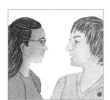

66 *I am concerned about Jim M. He said the other day that he was nauseated, and then again today. He does not talk very often, and rarely does he mention when he is uncomfortable. He is not able to answer any of the questions about the nausea. There is no record that he received any medications when he was nauseated a few days ago. His bowel movements are normal. He moves and transfers the same as before. His eating patterns have changed. He only eats little amounts and no snacks. This is a change for him. Jim's family is concerned. They noticed he was not eating, but did not know about the nausea. I gave him clear soup for lunch. Can you please see him?* 99

Pain

I remember a woman I cared for almost 30 years ago in a small-town hospital. Lying at the far end of the hall in a two-bed room, she would call out, "Nurse … Nurse … help me … Nurse …" and after a while, she would call out, "God, God, God … help me God." When I look back all these years later, I can still recall her name and can remember walking into her room, not knowing what to do or how to help. In retrospect, I think that she received acetaminophen a few times a day, but I am sure that she did not get anything else for her pain. My memory of her still haunts me, and I regret not having been a better support to her.

Pain is a signal sent to the brain that indicates that tissue or nerve damage is occurring. Pain is a common symptom of dying because the dying process involves progressive tissue damage. Sadly, pain is still one of the most feared symptoms people associate with dying.

Although tissue damage causes physical pain, physical pain is also a whole person experience. Physical pain affects the emotional, spiritual, and social parts of a person, and they affect physical pain. Untreated pain can result in depression, decreased mobility, decreased socialization, and sleep disturbances. When integrating a palliative approach, PSWs work with the whole person to manage pain.

Physical pain is a whole body experience that affects and is affected by emotional, spiritual and social parts of the person

Elderly people commonly have pain and many will have more than one source of pain. For the elderly, most pain is associated with musculoskeletal problems such as arthritis. Nerve pain can also result from diabetes, trauma, and amputation. Cancer can cause a variety of organ, muscle, bone, and nerve pain. The elderly are at highest risk for unrecognized pain and undertreatment of pain because they may not report their pain or, due to cognitive impairment, may not be able to report their pain.

Good pain management requires a team approach, and PSWs are invaluable resources in helping to gather information, identify comfort measures, and provide support. Your input helps the team fine-tune the medications used to help people achieve their goals for pain management.

Gathering Information

PSWs spend significant time providing care and therefore generally are familiar with the person's usual behaviour. This knowledge can help you identify early signs of discomfort when you are observing the person.

Observing

Often a person's behaviour changes even before they talk about pain. Therefore, caregivers who know a person's usual behaviour, who know what is normal and meaningful for the person, will be best at identifying changes that could indicate

Knowing a person's normal behaviour will help identify pain behaviours

pain. They will be able to detect early signs, and observe and report behavioural changes that may indicate untreated pain. This is especially important when people cannot speak about their pain, such as those who are cognitively impaired or not responsive, and/or those who do not speak English. It is helpful to ask the question, "I wonder what this behaviour is telling me about pain?"

Consider untreated pain when observing these behaviours

As a PSW, you might suspect untreated pain after observing in the person changes in any of the following:

- Behaviour, such as
  - Resistance to their usual care or activities
  - Not wanting to move certain body parts
  - Restricting overall movement
  - Decreasing participation in usual activities
- Function, such as
  - Increased distraction
  - Increased agitation
  - Restlessness or fidgeting
  - Rocking or pacing
- Posture, such as
  - Guarding
  - Holding their breath
  - Bracing
- Vocal and facial expressions, such as
  - Negative vocalizations like sighing, moaning, swearing, or grunting
  - Noisy breathing
  - Rapid respirations
  - Calling out for help
  - Facial expressions that show sadness, fatigue, or fright
  - Furrowed brow, squinting, clenched jaw, or grimacing

When you notice changes such as these, record them, describing how they are changes from this person's normal behaviour. If possible, ask the person questions to gather information about what may be causing such changes. Report your observations to the nurse.

I give morning care to a woman with advanced dementia. One morning I lifted her arm to wash her armpit and she pulled her arm away sharply, grimaced, moaned, and struck me with her other hand.

I wondered, "What is her behaviour telling me? Maybe her shoulder is sore and it hurts when I move it." I reported this to the nurse, and we discussed a few options to improve the resident's comfort.

Our plan: Tomorrow I will wait for one hour after she receives her morning pain medication before bathing her. I will wash her armpit without lifting her arm so high. And I will try putting a looser-fitting shirt on her. I will then report back to the nurse and discuss next steps. I will also watch the person I am caring for closely and see if there are other activities that seem to be causing her pain. Then the nurse can talk to the doctor if the medication needs to be increased.

PSWs use the Pain Assessment in Advanced Dementia (PAINAD) Scale[12] when caring for people who are cognitively impaired or unable to respond verbally. In using the PAINAD tool, the caregiver observes the person and assigns a score between 0 and 2 for five pain indicators/behaviours. The scores are added together for a final tally. It indicates whether a person's behaviour might be indicating pain, with higher scores more confidently indicating pain. Scores *do not* reflect the severity of pain, only the presence or absence of pain. When you use a tool like the PAINAD Scale repeatedly, changes in the person's status will be noticeable.

Pain Assessment in Advanced Dementia (PAINAD) Scale

	0	1	2	Score
Breathing Independent of vocalization	Normal	Occasional laboured breathing. Short period of hyperventilation	Noisy labored breathing. Long period of hyperventilation. Cheyne-stokes respirations.	
Negative Vocalization	None	Occasional moan or groan. Low level speech with a negative or disapproving quality	Repeated troubled calling out. Loud moaning or groaning. Crying.	
Facial Expression	Smiling, or inexpressive	Sad. Frightened. Frown.	Facial grimacing	
Body Language	Relaxed	Tense. Distressed pacing. Fidgeting.	Rigid. Fists clenched, knees pulled up. Pulling or pushing away. Striking out.	
Consolability	No need to console	Distracted or reassured by voice or touch	Unable to console, distract or reassure	
			TOTAL	

---

12 V. Warden, A.C. Hurley, and L. Volicer, "Development and Psychometric Evaluation of the Pain Assessment in Advanced Dementia (PAINAD) Scale," *Journal of the American Medical Directors Association* 4, no. 1 (2003): 9–15.

Observing to identify sources of pain

As you provide care, be alert for changes in the person's appearance, such as areas with redness, bruising, or swelling or areas that are warm. They may indicate a source of pain. Record these potential pain sources and report them to the nurse.

Asking questions

Margot McCaffery, an expert in the subject of pain, popularized the key principle in understanding a person's pain: "Pain is whatever the person says it is." An observer does not need to judge whether the pain is as severe or is more severe than reported.

1. Adapt the List of Sample Questions
2. Record
3. Report

You can adapt the questions in the List of Sample Questions to create your own questions to use in exploring and developing an understanding of the person's pain. Report your observations and preliminary information to the nurse. When a person's needs are urgent, and if the nurse or health care team is not available, proceed by asking detailed questions, such as in the examples below, to gather information that will help inform the nurse.[13]

> ***Are you in pain?*** *Do you have pain? Do you have any areas that hurt or are sore, tight, or uncomfortable?*

If a person is not fluent in English, it will be important to have a family member, community member, or friend available to translate. Ask them to write down a few words that mean "pain" or "discomfort" in the person's language for you to use at times when a translator is not available.

> ***When did the pain start?*** *Is this a new pain? Is it an increase in a pain that has been there for a while? When did the pain increase?*

> ***Where is the pain?*** *Can you tell me where your pain is? Can you point to it? Can you show me on this Body Map? Do you have pain in other areas? Do you have more than one pain?*

13 Remember that the person (and family) may be tired from answering questions. If it is inappropriate to ask further questions, provide the nurse with information based on your observations. You could say, "This is what I observed." Your observations and clear communication will help the nurse understand the importance and the urgency of your request.

Where is the pain?—using a Body Map to identify the location of pain

The Body Map not only helps the health care team learn more about a person's pain, but may also help people who struggle to tell about their pain. People with mild or moderate cognitive impairment may be able to use the body map to give information.

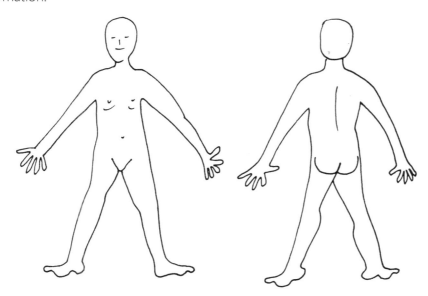

Provide the person with a Body Map and a pen or pencil. Ask them to draw on the map where they feel their pain. If their vision is compromised, you may want to enlarge the map. If the person is unable to use a pencil or pen, they may be able to point to the areas where they feel pain.

What does the pain feel like? *Can you describe your pain?*

People may describe their pain as burning, throbbing, tingling, aching, dull, sharp, stabbing, deep, cramping, coming and going, or electrical. The words the person uses will help the health care team identify the cause of and best treatment for the pain.

Pain can be described with many different words

Can you rate the pain on a scale? *Can you rate your pain on a scale of 0 to 10, in which 0 means no pain and 10 means the worst pain you can imagine?*

People may find it difficult to rate their pain. For some it may be the first time they have thought of pain in terms of a scale. Reassure the person that there is no right or wrong answer.

If a person is unable or unwilling to assign a number to their pain, you could ask them to describe it in words instead:

People may want to rate their pain with numbers or with words

Can you rate this pain as being mild, moderate, strong, or intense or severe?

Can you tell me if this is a small pain, a medium pain, or a big pain?

On occasion, the family may feel that their loved one's pain rating is not accurate.

My husband is very strong and does not like to talk about pain, so he says it is 3 out of 10, but that really means that it is more like a 6 out of 10.

This type of insight helps caregivers understand any hidden meaning in a person's communication. Record and report both the person's and the family members' comments. It may also help to use the person's own words, such as "discomfort" rather than "pain."

What makes the pain worse? What makes it better? *Is there anything that makes you more uncomfortable? Is there anything that makes you feel better, that decreases the pain, or that distracts you from feeling the pain?*

Answers to these questions help the health care team identify the best way to help. This information also informs the PSW about ways to adapt care for the person.

What can I do to be helpful? *Considering that you are so uncomfortable, how can we change plans for caregiving this morning, to get you more comfortable before I help you with your bath?*

"What can I do to be helpful?" is such a great question! Today, right now, what can you do to help the person in your care?

Your observations will be needed if the person or family cannot respond to the questions

If the person or their family cannot respond to questions, you will need to observe the person and communicate your observations to the nurse.

Reflection Activity on Different Types of Pain

Pain is produced through a number of different pathways in the body, each pathway producing different sensations. Reflect on a pain you experienced and describe the sensations. How do these pains differ?

- A mild toothache
- A muscle sprain
- A broken bone

- An episode of constipation
- The experience of childbirth
- The experience of passing a kidney stone

- A cold sore
- An episode of shingles
- A sunburn

As you consider these pains, you may notice how different each one is.

Pain comes from different types of body tissue, which is why each pain feels different.

How would you describe your experiences with pain?

The pain of a broken bone and a mild toothache may both involve localized aching pain from the bone and muscle. The person may describe their pain as deep, aching, penetrating, or probing. If the pain is untreated, it may spread to other areas.

Visceral pain comes from the organs, such as the heart, intestines, or liver. The pain may be local, it may seem to move around, or it may refer to another area of the body. Abdominal pain is often described as cramping, colicky, and intermittent, and is often associated with constipation. The pain comes in surges and may seem to move around.

Pain associated with a sunburn, a cold sore, or shingles involves the nerves. When this type of pain occurs, the skin is more sensitive than normal. Stimulation or touch that would not normally hurt may be really painful. This pain is caused by an "unhappy nerve" and is often a shooting pain, or the pain grabs the person instantly. Such pain is unpredictable. Neuropathic pain may be described as burning, itching, numbness, shooting, icy cold, "pins and needles," or like an electrical jolt. It usually follows a distinct pattern along a nerve pathway and may be continuous or intermittent.

It is possible to have pain that is a combination of the different types of pain. For example, a person with a toothache might have the constant aching, throbbing originating in the muscle and bone, and nerve pain causing severe sensitivity to heat, cold, or pressure.

People may also have several different types of pain caused by their illness and/or treatment for it.

Annette is one of the ladies on our unit. She often tries to leave the building. She paces and rattles the doors. One day she became more agitated. She started pacing faster and rattling the doors harder. I was less able to redirect her. I asked her if she was having pain. She nodded. She rubbed her back. I gave her a warm flannel to wrap around her shoulders while she was walking. I told the physiotherapist. He ordered an X-ray of her back. The X-ray showed a new compression fracture (broken bone) in Annette's back. That was what was causing increased pain and agitated behaviour. The nurse spoke with the doctor. The doctor increased the pain medications. After that Annette was much calmer; the pacing and rattling behaviours decreased.

Comfort Measures

Individualize comfort measures to this person at this time.

As a PSW, you can create a relaxing environment, reposition the person to provide support and comfort, use music or other distractions to decrease the perception of pain, and provide gentle touch to reduce discomfort. You can use comfort basket items to individualize care to the person's needs. Information gathered when a person is comfortable may help guide you in deciding which comfort measures to use when they are in pain. Remember that what works one day may not work another day. Invite the family to participate in assessing, sharing information, and offering comfort. Respect the dying person and individualize the care!

Preventive

Various ways in which you can help prevent pain are discussed below.

Creating a relaxing pace for daily activities
A person's sensation of pain often increases with stress. Therefore, create a daily plan that encourages an unhurried approach to daily activities.

Planning activities for times when the pain medication is most effective
Plan to do activities that may cause discomfort at a time when the person has the best pain relief in place. For example, if the person experiences some discomfort when being bathed, then plan to bathe the person about an hour after they receive pain medication.

Positioning for comfort

Prevent skin breakdown and ulceration by ensuring a smooth, clean, dry, and wrinkle free surface wherever the person is sitting or lying down. This is especially important for people who are less mobile and are unable to reposition themselves.

Checking mobility aids for safety

When people need to use a wheelchair for a limited time, they may borrow one that does not fit their body. Ensure that mobility aids are safe by checking the following:

- The fit of the wheelchair. Ensure that it does not put pressure on the person's arms, hips, heels, and calves, and that the person can use the footrests comfortably.
- The comfort of the seat. Ensure that the cushion is properly inflated and the pillow is positioned with the bowl in back and the bump in front, between the legs. When the person is not able to sit upright and remain centred on their own, they may benefit from having a wheelchair that tilts back (in such cases, consult with a rehabilitation professional). It may be helpful to have a physiotherapist or occupational therapist consult about what seating would be best for the person. Suggest a consult if the person
  - Squirms constantly in the wheelchair
  - Needs repositioning every 30 minutes
  - Has a pressure ulcer

Supporting the neck

Supporting the neck and head can provide comfort and enhance a person's feeling of security. Gently slide a soft pillow under the person's head and neck. Tug the pillow down to their shoulders so that it encircles their neck.

Repositioning the person slightly after raising the head of the bed

Make sure the person is high in the bed before raising the head of the bed. Once you have raised it, face the person and lean toward them with arms outstretched, putting your arms around the person as though you were going to hug them. Place your hands behind their shoulder blades, lift gently, and bring their entire body forward slightly. Lay the person back against the bed. This very simple procedure helps realign their back and their clothing. It may sound simple, but when people cannot reposition themselves, it is wonderful when their caregiver employs this strategy. Try it!

Taking pressure off the coccyx when the person is sitting or lying

When a person has a pressure ulcer or discomfort on the coccyx, place a soft thin pillow under the fleshy part of the buttock to reposition the person slightly. This will take some weight off the tailbone.

Elevating swollen lower limbs

When a person has swollen feet or lower legs, elevate the foot of the bed. Insert a few folded blankets or a thin pillow under the foot of the bed between the mattress and the bed frame. Over a period of eight hours, the swelling should decrease. This will improve comfort and reduce risk of pressure ulcers in the heels.

Turning a person in stages through the night

Before turning a person, remove the pillows. Replace them after the turn.

Repositioning regularly improves comfort

Over the course of a night, you can gradually move a person from one side to their other side with small movements every few hours. Repositioning every few hours reduces the risk of pressure ulcers. Slight adjustments mean that the person is not lying on the same pressure points. For instance, the person may start the night far over on their right side and then slowly, over a few turns, be closer to lying on their back. From there, turn the person to their left side. Then, using small adjustments over the next few turns, adjust until the person is nearly on their back again. Small adjustments make it possible to turn a sleeping person while disturbing them as little as possible.

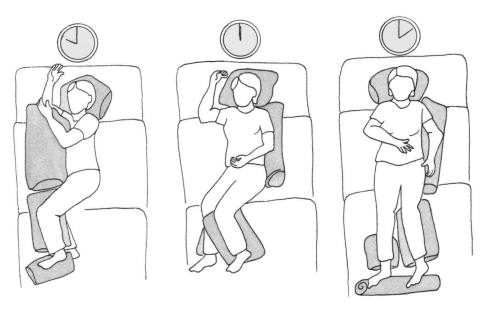

Laying the person on their side

These are the steps in laying a person on their side:
1. Roll the person onto one side. Place a pillow behind the back, being careful to remove wrinkles in bedclothes and sleepwear.
2. Gently grasp the shoulder blade the person is lying on and pull the arm forward toward you.
3. Move their top leg forward and bend the knee. Position a pillow between the legs, supporting the lower part of the legs.
4. Shift their pelvis forward slightly by pulling the slider sheet and hips toward you.
5. Position a pillow under the upper arm.
6. Reposition the pillow between the legs to decrease pressure on the ankle joints.

Protecting the skin before turning the person

Before turning a person, gently stroke or massage the skin on the side they will be lying on. Light massage will improve blood flow and reduce skin breakdown. After turning the person, do not touch or massage the newly exposed skin on which they have lain. The oxygen-deprived tissues are very susceptible to damage.

Position and reposition the person for comfort. Bed-bound and mobility-limited people are at high risk for pressure ulcers. Reposition the person every two to four hours to reduce the risk of pressure ulcers.

In the moment

Distracting for comfort

> Distracting a person can decrease their pain for a short time. A person can be distracted by chatting while visiting, having stories told to them, reminiscing, laughing, being with a pet, watching TV or videos, reading, or breathing fresh air. Explore which distractions might work best for the person in your care. As with any of the comfort measures, individualize the care. What might distract someone from their pain might cause another person to feel more pain!

Distracting a person can provide comfort for a short time. Consider this strategy when a person is waiting for a pain medication to take effect or is in the midst of a painful procedure. Distraction might help during a five-minute dressing change that usually causes the person discomfort or when they do not want medication or extra medication.

Distraction and relaxation measures are excellent short term comfort measures

Relaxing for comfort

Relaxation strategies such as massage, guided imagery, breathing exercises, and music care can decrease the sensation of pain, as well as improve the effectiveness of medications. Guided imagery can help a person relax until the regular dose or breakthrough dose takes effect.

Guided Imagery

When you provide care for someone, talk with the person about the activities they love, the places they enjoy, their favourite place to sit and relax … You might ask questions such as these:

What is your favourite place? The cottage? What time of year? What time of day? Where do you like to sit? What does the ground feel like? What do see? What do you feel? What do you smell? What do you hear?

When the person is uncomfortable, for example, while waiting for pain medication to take effect, you might suggest that they try to imagine relaxing in their favourite place.

Use the images shared by the dying person to create a guided imagery.

You might say something like this:

While the medication takes effect, close your eyes and think for a few minutes about that favourite spot of yours at the cottage. Imagine that you are sitting on your favourite rock overlooking the lake. It is late summer. The grasses are dry, and you can feel the dry prickly grasses with your fingers. The ground is hard beneath you. You are leaning back against another rock, warmed by the sun. The breeze off the water smells fresh. The grasses smell warm and dry, that smell of late summer. You look across the lake and see your favourite tree, the one you like to climb. You can hear the birds, and you especially love those birds that perch on the trees nearby. Breathe the fresh air. Take it in gently. Then let your breath out. Relax and enjoy the summer warmth, the warm flannel, and rest for a bit …

Comfort measures that stimulate
- warm flannel
- heat
- cooling or ice
- gentle massage

Stimulating for comfort

Warm flannels, heated beanbags, fresh cool cloths, frozen compresses, or creamy lotions applied with a gentle but firm touch can stimulate the senses and help the mind focus on something other than pain.

Place a warm flannel between the person and their blankets, folded behind their back, or simply over the legs.

Sometimes gentle stimulation in one area can decrease the sensation of pain in another. Consider applying gentle but firm touch on the side of the body opposite from where they feel pain.

Gentle massage may be soothing, but care should be taken to avoid touching or massaging sensitive or painful areas. Check your employer's policies and guidelines about the type of touch and massage you are permitted to offer.

Before using these comfort measures, remember to ask the person whether they would like you to.

For the family

Invite the family to participate in providing comfort. Care provided by family can be particularly effective at soothing a person. It also comforts the family because they feel helpful and involved. Some family members may feel completely comfortable participating in the person's caregiving, or they may need prompting or guidance to get started. You might make suggestions like this:

> *I heard you say that you would like to give your mom mouth care but don't know how to do that. Would it be helpful if I showed you how to freshen her mouth?*

Comfort measures provided by family can sooth the person and the family

Wheelchair massage

A person sitting in a wheelchair can become quite stiff even after a short time. People with normal mobility maintain their comfort by constantly changing their posture and position in multiple little ways. People with limited mobility cannot make these little adjustments and become uncomfortable as time passes. Therefore, it may be soothing for a person with limited mobility who is in a wheelchair for an extended time to have a wheelchair massage. This may not be in the scope of the PSW's practice and is suggested here as a comfort strategy that family can provide.

These are directions for giving a wheelchair massage:
- Slip your hands between the person's body and the chair.
- While resting the back of the hand against the chair, apply gentle pressure with curved fingers and massage or press
  - on the back
  - under the legs
  - under the hips

Encourage family to do those things that the person enjoyed doing before becoming ill. A person may want their loved one to hold or snuggle them. The person may appreciate your help in getting the family member snuggled comfortably and safely in the bed. The side bar may help to hold the second person safely in bed.

Medications and Treatments

A number of medications can be used to help manage pain. The principles of palliation and principles of using medications to manage symptoms were presented at the beginning of Chapter 4 because they apply to managing all of the symptoms discussed in the chapter. It is *essential* that you review those principles again as you study this section about pain management.

Additional information about medications used to manage pain is provided in the appendix. Depending on your scope of practice, you may not need to know all of the additional information, but knowing the basics and familiarizing yourself with the content in appendix A may be helpful.

Below are a few key messages about medication used for pain management:
- Pain medication is divided into two categories, analgesics and adjuvant analgesics.
- Analgesics are medications that specifically work to reduce pain.
- Analgesics are divided into two groups, opioid and non-opioid analgesics.
  - Opioids include morphine, hydromorphone, oxycodone, fentanyl, sufenta, codeine, and so on.
  - Non-opioids include acetaminophen and ibuprofen.
- Adjuvant medications may be used to treat another symptom but their secondary effect is pain relief.
  - Adjuvant medications include steroids, non-steroidal antinflammatories, anticonvulsants, antispasmodics, antidepressants, and antibiotics.
- The principles of palliation (page 58) and principles of using medications to manage symptoms (page 58) should be understood and followed.

If you are working with people who experience pain, ensure that you are familiar with the content in appendix A, the principles for using opioids to manage pain, the fears and misconceptions about opioids, and the common side effects of opioids. Be familiar with questions you can ask to gather information about pain, the importance of following up after medication is administered, and the importance of recording and reporting initially and during the follow-up.

- Gather information
- Follow up after medications
- Record
- Report

There are many types of treatment for pain. The ideal treatment choice is the one that works for the person in pain and helps them meet their goals. Examples of non-invasive treatments are physiotherapy, massage therapy, acupuncture, guided imagery, and meditation. Invasive treatments include surgery, nerve blocks, radiation therapy, and chemotherapy.

The health care team consults with the person to determine the most appropriate treatment, given the person's goals of care.

Sample Report

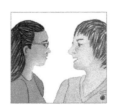

66 *I just went to provide care for Mrs. C. She was in her recliner, did not want to have her bath, was holding tight to a pillow, and was not chatting as she usually does. I asked is she was having pain, and she nodded yes. I showed her the body map and she pointed to the right leg and hip. She did have some pain yesterday according to the chart. I don't know if she had any medication or if the pain settled. When I have seen her with this pain in her leg and hip, I normally help reposition her and put on her favourite music, and the nurse gives her a breakthrough medication. Today I repositioned her, am playing the music she likes, and wonder if you [the nurse] can see her about the medication. When she is more settled, then I can help her with her bath.* 99

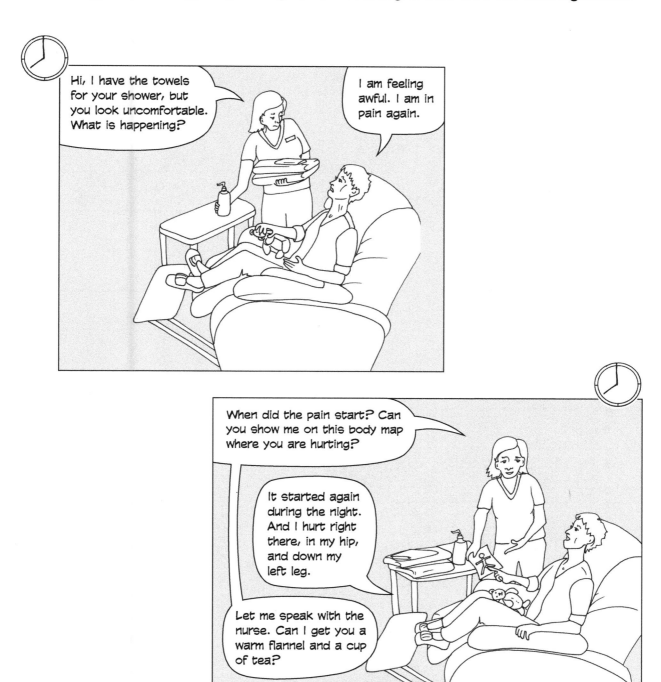

continued on page 116 ...

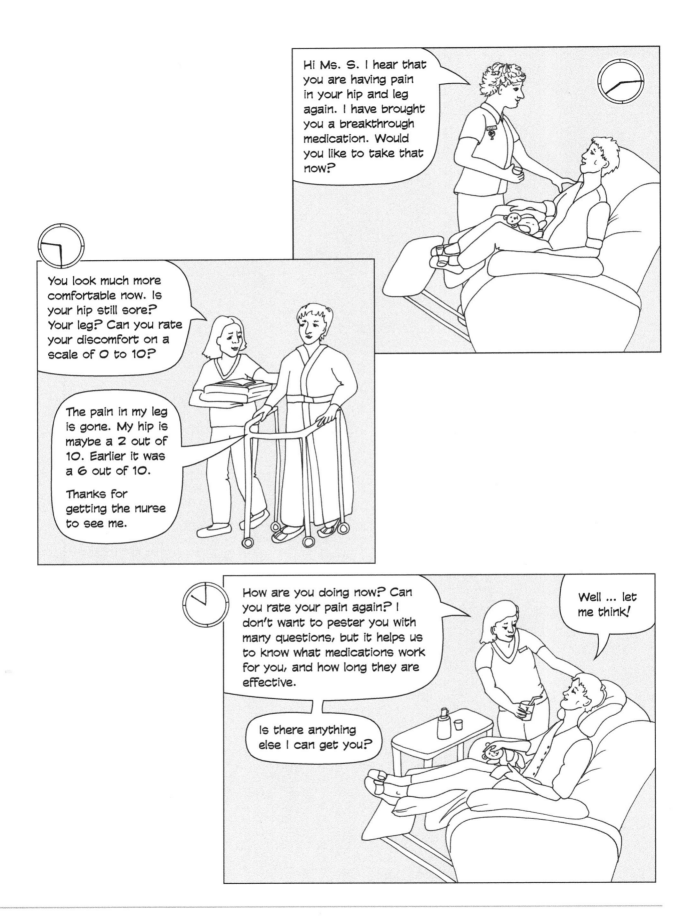

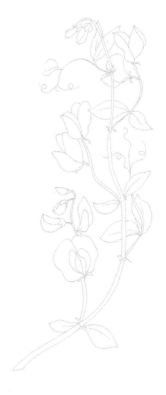

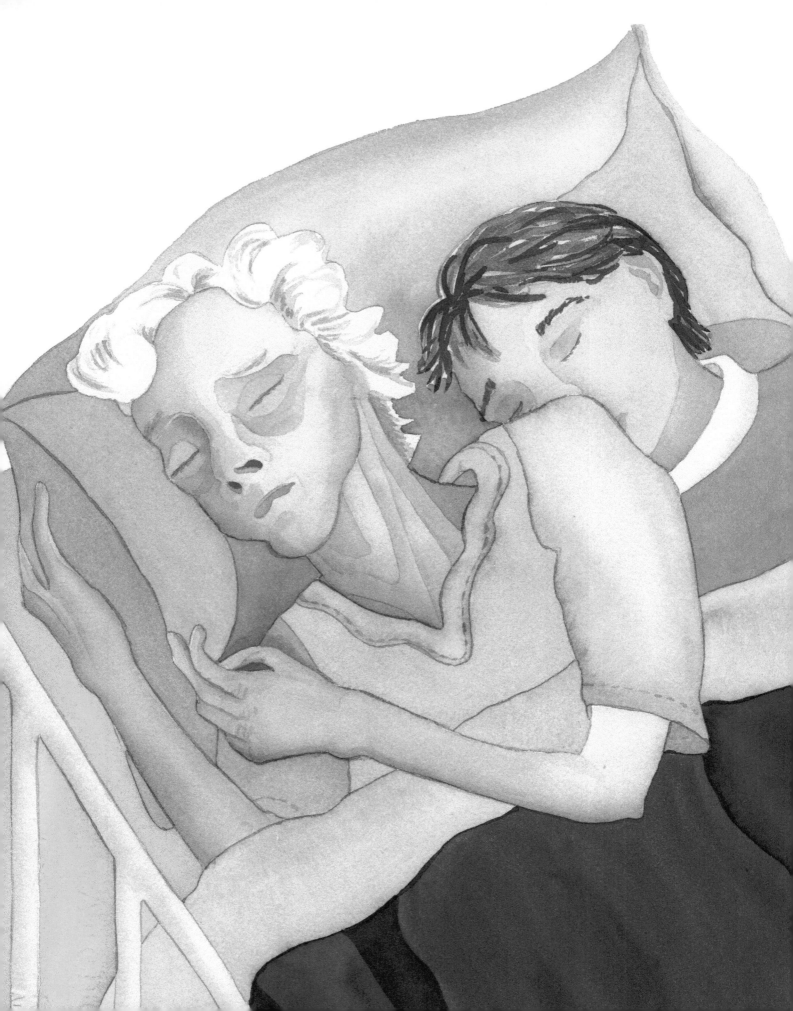

5

Providing Psychosocial Care

The word "psychosocial" refers to the emotional, intellectual, spiritual, interpersonal, and cultural aspects of a person. Simply said, it means "everything except the physical." In this text, physical symptoms and psychosocial issues are addressed in separate chapters. However, people do not experience life in an unconnected or compartmentalized way. Human beings are holistic. All physical symptoms have emotional implications, and emotions, such as grief, can actually change a person physically at the cellular level. It is important to remember the holistic approach. The person is more than their illness, more than the sum of their body parts, and more than their emotional reaction to death, dying, loss, and grief.

Transitions at any time of life can be complex. Transitions that include illness, discomfort, decline in functioning and health, uncertainty, and lack of control are challenging. The focus of this chapter is on providing psychosocial support for the person and family experiencing transitions, uncertainty, loss, and grief. Advance care planning is discussed as a way to help people direct their future care now in case they become unable to later.

I acknowledge that the strategies provided here focus more on providing emotional support than on providing social, intellectual, interpersonal, or spiritual support. And yet, the emotional support PSWs provide by its very nature influences and affects those other types of support. I hope that I can offer you ideas and inspiration for being with and responding to those you care for in a way that creates a nurturing, safe place that will help the person and the family grow, even as the person is dying.

Transitions

Supporting through Periods of Decline

Three Victoria Hospice counsellors, Moira Cairns, Marney Thompson, and Wendy Wainwright, wrote a book titled *Transitions in Dying and Bereavement: A Psychosocial Guide for Hospice and Palliative Care*. In it they identify psychosocial issues that commonly occur as a person's level of functioning decreases, as indicated by a score on the Palliative Performance Scale (PPS) (see page 51). Key times of transition include those of the initial diagnosis and the recurrence or progression of disease, the time when illness dominates, the time when the person becomes totally bed bound, and the period of watching and waiting as death becomes imminent.

PPS 100%–90%

Disease may be diagnosed in a person when their score on the PPS is between 100% and 90%. At this time, the person and their family struggle to understand the illness and make decisions about treatment. The person may then recover and return to their previous activities of daily life. As a PSW, you may care for such people while they are in hospital to have tests, receive a diagnosis, or undergo treatment. The physician, counsellor, and nurse will provide information to help the person make decisions about treatment. You can provide emotional support as you listen to their fears, concerns, and questions about treatment, and you can communicate with the team as needed. You can also assure the person that making decisions is difficult and offer support for the decisions made.

PPS 80%–70%

The disease may reoccur or, in the case of chronic illness, not respond to treatment, and the person may be readmitted to hospital. At this point, the person has a PPS score between 80% and 70%. The authors of *Transitions in Dying and Bereavement* call this "the path not chosen." And so it is. The person had hoped for a cure, and now the disease has raised its head once again. The person is in a state of limbo. They are neither healthy nor dying and may feel disconnected from others. As a PSW, you can provide support when you ask open-ended questions and listen while the person reflects on their situation.

PPS 60%–50%

When a person has a PPS score between 60% and 50%, the disease is extensive. It is advanced and a cure is not possible. The person can no longer ignore the illness. Fatigue and weakness often mean that the person is no longer able to work or participate in their hobbies, and they may spend most of their time sitting or lying down. The person and their family need to adjust their roles and responsibilities. The person may transition from receiving acute curative treatments to comforts provided in a hospice palliative care approach. This may include registration with a hospice program. You can provide emotional support when you acknowledge the many losses, the different grieving experiences and styles of family members, and the challenges that may occur between family members.

PPS 40%–30%

A person with a PPS score between 40% and 30% is weaker and often very tired, and becomes unable to provide self-care. Initially the person may still want to get out of bed, and if the person has delirium or is restless, this period can be one of intense caregiving and supporting of the family. Once the person is in bed full-time, the work of caregiving may be a bit less stressful. This may be a difficult time for the dying person who is no longer independent. The person and their family redefine roles and responsibilities once again. This is often the time when the PSW becomes involved in providing full-time personal care. In the home setting, you help the person and their family as you organize new routines for personal care. In a long-term care facility, on the person's first day you welcome the person to their new home, as well as welcome the family, and provide supports for what is often a most difficult day. In addition to this, you provide support when you listen to the person's story, help them to remember their strengths, and identify local resources and contact numbers.

When the person's score on the PPS descends to between 20% and 10%, the person becomes less alert, is less responsive, and in many ways disconnects from the living. As a PSW, you can provide psychosocial support for the dying person by offering your presence, being with the person and the family, talking with the person as though they were still able to hear you, coaching the person, and if appropriate, gently explaining what is happening.

The family transitions at this point from "doing for" to "being with." As a PSW, you can nurture and support the family by providing nourishment, responding to questions, communicating with the nurse, providing information brochures, and being a reassuring presence. (See Chapter 6 for further information about last days and hours.)

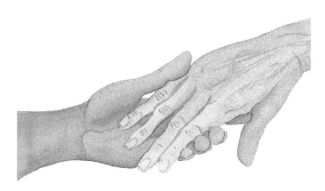

Sharing Information

Information helps people to make decisions

One reason that the transitions in dying are difficult is because of uncertainty. It is helpful for people to know what to expect, what resources are available, what changes might occur, and whom to contact with questions or concerns when a crisis occurs. When people have information, they are more able to make informed decisions, participate in care planning, and access the health care team more effectively as needs arise.

For information sharing to be effective, it is helpful to know what kind of information the person and their family prefer and what type of materials they find easiest to understand.

I am reminded of the Dr. Seuss children's book *Green Eggs and Ham*. In the book, Sam is trying to get an unnamed character to taste green eggs and ham. The unnamed character responds, "I do not like green eggs and ham. I do not like them, Sam-I-Am." This continues as Sam tries to get him to eat green eggs and ham in many locations with several different animals. And the unnamed character keeps trying to explain to Sam that he does not like them, will not like them. He repeats, "I would not like them here or there. I would not like them anywhere!" Finally, he tries the food and he likes it after all, and responds, "I do so like green eggs and ham. Thank you. Thank you, Sam-I-Am."

Like the character who does not want to try green eggs and ham, most people do not really want to know about dying. And when people do need the information, they may not want it or know how helpful it is. And so it is the PSW's job to find out how to make this information palatable, digestible, and easy to understand. As in *Green Eggs and Ham*, when people get the information, they often express deep appreciation for the information and how helpful it is.

Remember to listen for preferences in how a family learns information

The health care team can be helpful by sharing information with the person and their family in a way that works for them:
- Information should be
  - Consistent—it is a good thing to hear someone say, "You all say the same thing."
  - Delivered with compassion
  - Shared regularly as needed, and repeated if necessary
- The information should be offered in a way compatible with the preferred style of learning of the person and family.
  - Some people will want a lot of information; others will want only a small amount on a need-to-know basis.
  - Some people will want the textbook version; others will want brochures, simple YouTube videos, or written directions.

The following two stories show how two people have completely different preferences for how much information they want to receive.

Shared information
needs to be
- consistent
- shared with
  compassion
- shared regularly

"Do you want information?" I asked him.

"Well, if I am dying tomorrow, I want to know."

"Do you want information?" I asked him.

"No, like, if I am … If I am … you know, if I am going [pointing upwards], I don't want to know."

"Can I talk with your wife about what is happening?"

"Yes, you can talk with her, but I don't want to talk about it."

As a PSW, you provide support when you do the following:
- Listen to the person and empathize with them about their concerns and questions, and connect with the appropriate health care team member as necessary.

Supporting during
transitions includes:
- listening
- empathizing
- explaining
- connecting with the
  health care team

  Those are excellent questions about what to expect in the coming days and weeks. I encourage you to talk with the doctor or the nurse about those questions. I can ask the nurse to see you, and I can give you the phone number to make an appointment with your husband's physician. Would that be helpful?

- Communicate when people do not understand information that has been shared with them.

  Mrs. Singh is confused about the medications. This morning she said, "I don't know when I am supposed to give these pills. The nurse showed me, but I don't understand. I don't know what to do." Can you [the nurse] please see her?

- Identify the type of learning strategies that the person and family prefer to use and share that information with health care team.

Inform the health
care team when you
suspect that the
person or family do
not understand the
information provided

  The brother uses the Internet to read about the disease. He likes lots of details and scientific information. The rest of the family really likes the brochures you gave them.

- Ensure that the person and family know how to contact the health care team at any time of the day or week.

  Do you have the numbers to phone if you need help in the middle of the night? May I post that information on the fridge?

- Work with the health care team to identify other people who can provide support to the person and family if they have no one to call at night.

The next section discusses what can be expected for people who are dying with dementia. Relatively little is known about dying with dementia, so talking about what is known is helpful.

Common questions about dying with dementia

The Dementia Difference: Integrating a Palliative Approach in Caring for People with Dementia[1]

Caring for someone dying with dementia has a few unique challenges: the person is unable to participate in decision making, there are many uncertainties, and the family may be exhausted after extended periods of caregiving.

These are some of the questions frequently asked about the uncertainties that relate to people dying with dementia:

- When will death occur?

    I don't know how long he has. Do I need to keep up my energy for months or years?

- What will the trajectory look like?

    What can I anticipate? What is going to happen?

- What will death will look like?

    Will he be peaceful? Will he die suddenly? Will I know when death is going to happen?

- What other illnesses will contribute to dying?

    Does it matter that he also has diabetes and kidney failure?

- What is going to happen next?

    When she eats her dinner, I wonder if she is getting better. When she has a bad day, I wonder if she is dying. Tonight she ate her dinner. Is she getting better?

---

1 Thanks to Broadmead Care Society in Victoria, BC, for the opportunity to develop a staff-education workshop titled "The Dementia Difference: Integrating a Palliative Approach in Caring for People with Dementia, in 2007, revised in 2013.

It is important to not get stuck in the uncertainties and to remember the certainties that are known about people dying with dementia:

- The overall trajectory will be a decline.
  - There may be ups and downs, but overall, there is a decline.
  - A person with Alzheimer's type dementia will first lose skills associated with higher-level functioning, such a balancing a chequebook or following a recipe. Eventually the person will lose more basic skills, including doing self-care, dressing, and walking. Eventually people with this type of dementia will not be able to feed themselves, and if they live long enough, they will lose the ability to swallow, one of the most basic reflexive behaviours.
- Death is certain to occur.
  - It is easy to forget this reality when a person has declined slowly over so many years, when the person has improved in the past when they seemed to be dying, and when the person seems relatively stable now. Death is certain to occur.
- Comorbidities will affect the trajectory.
  - If a person is healthy other than having whatever is causing the dementia, they might live longer than a person who has a history of strokes, diabetes, cancer of a vital organ, and so on.
- Certain interventions, such as those below, are not effective in late-stage dementia:
  - Attempts at cardiopulmonary resuscitation
  - Gastric tubes, which *do not*
    - Increase survival
    - Reduce the risk of infection
    - Prevent aspiration
    - Improve functional status
    - Improve comfort
  - Transfers to hospital for intravenous antibiotics
    - IV antibiotics are no more effective than oral antibiotics for repeat infections in late-stage dementia. The body requires a functioning immune system for antibiotics to be effective.
    - Antibiotics are not essential for comfort in the last days.
- Several indicators often precede the actively dying phase for people dying with dementia. In the period before death, the person may
  - Have repeated infections
  - Have skin ulcers that do not heal
  - Have a significant decline in intake
  - Be unable to swallow
  - Increasingly sleep and withdraw from others

Certainties about dying with dementia

Indicators that precede active dying with dementia

See Chapter 6 for more information on last days and hours.

Supporting Choice, Control, and Independence

The dying person has little control over their disease, the progressive changes their body goes through, the health care system, the team, and the resources offered. At a time when control is minimal, it is helpful to allow and encourage the person to make whatever decisions are important to them. And at a time when normal routines are disrupted, it is helpful to maintain or restore a sense of normalcy.

As a PSW, you can provide support when you do the following:

Ways for PSWs to acknowledge and support choice and independence for the dying person

- Acknowledge the desire for independence.

  I know that you prefer to care for yourself. Is there anything I can do that would make receiving help more comfortable for you?

- Support independence when possible.

  It looks like you can wash yourself today. Let me know if you need any assistance.

  You seem a bit shaky. I wonder if I can do that for you today.

- Provide choice whenever possible.

  Would you like your bath before or after you have lunch?

- Communicate client choices and goals to the health care team.

  This morning Sabita told me that she does not want to go back to hospital and does not want more treatment. I hear that Sabita is scheduled for more treatments. Can you please meet with her?

- Maintain rituals.

  I understand you have a morning routine with your family. Would you prefer that I arrive later in the morning to provide care?

- Invite the person to determine the priorities.

  What can I do for you this morning so that you can save your energy for the things that are most important to you?

  Yesterday was very busy with friends coming to visit. In the evening you said that you were really wiped out. What is your preference for today? Would you like us to decrease the number of visitors or the length of their stay?

- Respect the person's right to choose or refuse treatment, to eat or not, to bathe or not.

  I hear you, and I respect your decision to choose whether or not to continue with treatment.

Supporting Hope

Hope is both fragile and resilient. Hope is not rational; it does not depend on statistics or facts.

A person who receives a diagnosis of a life-threatening illness may hope that the illness will not significantly affect their quality of life, that it will be curable, and that it will not cause their death. When the same person is told, "There is nothing more that we can do, and there is no cure available," they may maintain hope for a long life, even when they recognize that it would take a miracle to cure them.

Hope can help sustain a person's emotional well-being by allowing them to look forward to good things in the future. A dying person may say, "I hope I can go fishing next summer like I have done for 55 years!" even when they know they may not live through the next month.

It is not helpful to confront a person with the reality that they are dying. It would not be supportive to say, "Don't you understand? You will never be able to go fishing again." Neither would it be helpful to say, "Of course you'll be able to go fishing next summer. Just set your mind to it and think positive thoughts."

As a PSW, you can provide support when you
- Respond from a genuine but neutral place

   Wouldn't that be wonderful? I hope you get your wish. What else do you hope for?

- Respond to the feelings behind the hope

   It sounds like you loved fishing. Where was your favourite fishing hole? What is your favourite fishing story?

PSWs support hope by responding to the feelings behind the hope

Hope is always possible. Hope can change. When someone can no longer hope for a cure, it is possible to hope to see the next grandchild born, or to hope for a pain-free death, or to hope the family will be well supported following death.

> *Michelle had four hopes. She hoped to live until Christmas, to enjoy our trip to Hawaii in January, to have a birthday party for her nephew, and to make it to Easter. She got three out of four of her wishes.* —A.S.

Hope changes

Maintaining Family Relationships

My grandmother got really depressed when she was dying. It turns out that she did not like being in a back bedroom. She wanted to be in the living room to know what was happening. She wanted to give us her advice and tell us what to do. She wanted to make decisions still. Once we put her in the front room and she was part of the action, then she stopped being so sad.

Maintaining family relationships can be important to both the person and the family. In the story above, it is clear that the grandmother had a role that was important to her and did not want it to change. On the other hand, there are times when roles have to change, when the person is no longer able to contribute as they did before they were sick. It may be helpful to acknowledge the loss and explore what roles the person can continue to fill.

As a person declines, there are often medical equipment and supplies in the bedroom and throughout the house. You can provide support when you do the following to create a comfortable place where people can gather and be with the dying person:

Support family time by creating a comfortable place to gather and visit

- Strive to put away medical equipment and supplies after using them, and then clean up the surroundings so the environment is comfortable and fresh for the person and family
- Arrange the room so that family members can sit in chairs, lie on the bed, or stretch out on the floor so that both the person and the family can be comfortable
- Tailor your actions to the needs of the people involved

When a dying person is being cared for by others and people are coming and going from the room, it may be difficult for them to find space, time, and energy for intimacy and closeness. You may want to discuss this with the person and their family.

Remember that the person and their loved one may want time for intimacy and closeness

There are so many people coming and going. Do you want to have some space for just the two of you?

Sometimes people don't realize that there is room for two people on a hospital bed. Would you like your loved one to climb up here so you could both be comfortable?

If you would like some time to yourself, we could put a do-not-disturb sign on the door. How would that be?

Is there anything else that would be helpful?

Advance Care Planning – Having a Say through to Death

I have talked about the challenges of transition and uncertainty. Supportive strategies to help people cope with transitions and uncertainty include providing information and supporting choice and control. Advance Care Planning is the formal term for the very informal conversations that happen between the person and family and professionals to ensure that the dying person's hopes, fears, wishes, and priorities are honoured when the person is no longer able to direct their own care. It is the process that is used to help people "have their own say" through to death.

What Is Advance Care Planning?

Advance Care Planning is about the conversations that people have with loved ones and health care providers about their values, beliefs, and hopes. It is the process of planning for your care, in the event that you can no longer speak, make decisions, or direct your own care. The person and family gather medical information so that informed discussions about care can be made. An Advance Care Planning talk may include addressing concerns like these:

> When I think about death, I worry about … [being alone, not being able to breathe …].

> When I am nearing death, I want … [soft music playing, someone to hold my hand, a blessing by my priest …].

> When I am nearing death, I want my friends and family to remember … [I love you, I forgive you …].

In the Advance Care Plan, the person identifies which medical interventions they would like used or not used. The person may assign a Substitute Decision Maker (other terms are used across Canada to refer to the person who fills this role) to make decisions for them if they are no longer able to make their own decisions. It is recommended that the dying person assign a substitute decision maker.

The legal forms and documents relating to Advance Care Planning differ across Canada. It is important that people who want to write down their wishes and instructions or name a Substitute Decision Maker do so ahead of time on the appropriate provincial or territorial forms.

What is a Substitute Decision Maker?

A Substitute Decision Maker is chosen by the person or the health care team to speak on behalf of the person in the event that he or she is no longer able to direct his or her own care. The Substitute Decision Maker should know the person well, have had Advance Care Planning conversations with the person, and be willing to honour their wishes. In many provinces and territories, a person can legally appoint a Substitute Decision Maker while capable. If the person has not assigned a Substitute Decision Maker, the provincial government will have a legal process to identify one.

What is the role of the Substitute Decision Maker?

Ideally, the role of the Substitute Decision Maker is to be actively involved in the care of the dying person, perhaps accompany the person to medical appointments, and regularly engage in conversations with the person. When a Substitute Decision Maker is making health care decisions, they must be based on what the dying person wants, not based on what the Substitute Decision Maker would want for herself or himself. The Substitute Decision Maker's scope is restricted to health care decisions only and not, for example, financial decisions.

What is the role of the family in making decisions?

Families and close friends play an important role in a person's life. While one family member or friend may provide consent for a particular treatment, the remaining family members and friends will also have important information to share with the health care team. For instance, a cousin may know that in their last hours the person wanted a particular song playing in their room. Family members and friends should be encouraged to share and communicate this type of information.

Supporting the Advance Care Planning Process

You will understand the Advance Care Planning process much better and be prepared to help others if you go through it for yourself:
- Reflect on what is important to you as a person. What gives your life meaning? What gives you joy, strength, and support?
- Talk with a friend or colleague and share your thoughts.
- Record on paper what values or ideas you want your Substitute Decision Maker to consider if you were to become unable to speak for yourself.
- Who would you like to ask to be your substitute decision maker?

My daughter came to visit. I wanted to talk with her about what is important to me in my life and what I want as I age and when I am dying. I know that talking about this before I am sick is a good idea. But she just responded by saying, "Oh Mom, let's not talk about that today!" But she has been saying that for the last year!

Talking about Advance Care Plans might feel foreign for many people. In your work as a PSW, you can help people in their process when you do the following:
- Validate their desire to talk about their personal wishes and hopes.

I want to talk with my family about my illness, but they don't want to talk about it.

You might respond:

That must be hard. I wonder if someone from the health care team—the nurse, physician, or social worker—could talk with you more about this. Would it be all right if I mention that to the nurse? Or would you rather mention it yourself?

Remember to follow up on your next visit.

- Acknowledge the lack of interest in discussing end of life issues, and at the same time share a healthy attitude about Advance Care Planning conversations.

  I don't want to talk about all this sad stuff.

You might respond:

I hear you. It is not uncommon for people to postpone these conversations. But you know, I have listened to conversations that were definitely not *sad. It is really about you exploring who you are, what you care about, and what you want. It is about making a plan.*

- Encourage conversations about the goals of care.

  The nurse wants to know what I want done in the future as I get more sick, and as death becomes more imminent.

Encourage conversations around Advance Care Planning

You might respond:

How do you feel about having a conversation like that? When your kids come this weekend, do you think it might be possible to discuss it with them?

Do you need some help to find the words to open the conversation? (Communicate this information to the nurse.)

- Help the person learn about medical procedures.

  I don't understand what they are going to do tomorrow.

You might respond:

That must be a bit worrisome. Could you talk with the doctor or nurse about your questions? Sometimes it is hard to remember what you were going to ask when you get to an appointment. I'd be happy to help you write down your questions and concerns.

- Help the person think about what's right for them.

  I need more care and I don't want to burden my family.

You might respond:

> *That's a hard one. Can you tell me more?* (Follow up on the next visit. Talk this over with the nurse.)

- Help the person prepare to talk with the health care professionals about medication or treatment concerns.

> *I don't want to take all these medications.*

You might respond:

> *Sounds like you have had enough of taking pills. What's happening? Can you talk with your doctor or nurse about how you are feeling?*

Here's another example:

> *I'm so tired of dialysis.*

You might respond:

> *It's a tiring process isn't it? Can you tell me a little more about what you are thinking and feeling? Who have you talked with about this?*

PSWs can help people prepare for conversations with family and doctors

- Help the person record conversations.

> *Maybe you could write down some of these thoughts and questions so you can talk with your doctor and family. Would you like me to take notes during this conversation if no one else is available?*

- Encourage the person to talk with the health care professionals, and provide contact information. You might say things like this:

> *There are people who can help you talk with your daughter about this. Would you like to talk to one of the other members of the team?*

> *It sounds like you are clear on your goals. Can you talk with the nurse, physician, or social worker about this?*

Know the legal boundaries of your work as a caregiver

PSWs at work cannot

Sign documents, including wills, legal forms, or contracts
- Tell someone what they should or should not do or what treatments they should have
- Make recommendations for Advance Care Planning decisions

Muriel, aged 89, had been living in an assisted living facility for several years. Over that time her condition had slowly declined, although she still ate well and enjoyed a number of activities with friends. One day the PSW who was caring for her and knew her quite well said to Muriel, "You seem especially quiet today. Are you feeling okay?"

"Well," Muriel said, "my best friend Joan died unexpectedly last week, and it's really gotten me thinking about when I die and where I want to be buried. My children don't want to talk about it, but although I've lived out West for a long time, my heart is really on the prairies and I would like to buried there with the rest of my family."

The PSW responded, "Thank you for sharing that information with me. I think it's quite natural that your friend's death would get you thinking about what's important to you, and it sounds like it might be helpful to consider some ways to bring this subject up with your family. Would it be okay if I asked your nurse to let you know who might be the best person on the team to help you do that?"

"Thank you!" Muriel said. "I know I may have a lot of time before I die, but it would be such a relief to me to know that my family knew my wishes."

Loss and Grief

People experience **loss** when they are deprived of someone or something import-ant to them. **Grief** is a healthy and natural adaptive response to loss. People **grieve** when they lose someone or something that is important to them. **Grieving** is the process of adapting to the loss in the changed environment. Grieving is a whole person experience that includes the sorrow and suffering caused by the loss, as well as the personal growth and insight that people may experience after a loss. A pal-liative approach supports the dying person from the time of diagnosis through the dying process and care of the body following death. A palliative approach supports the family from time of diagnosis through time of death and through the grieving process.

Basic Truths about Loss and Grief

The facts about loss and grief

There are many theories about loss and grief. Models of grief have been developed, refined, and changed as new understanding develops. There are basic truths about loss and grief that all members of the health care team should understand:

- Loss is natural. Everyone experiences loss as part of being alive.
- People whose health is declining and who are dying experience multiple losses.
- Grief is a natural, healthy response to loss that helps people adapt to living in a changed world.
- Grief is a whole person experience.
- People grieve differently over time
- People grieve in different and unique ways.
- Denial can be an effective way to cope with overwhelming loss and grief.
- Hope is a wish for something that is important to the person.

Making Friends with Gone

(Most) all the food's been put away
A little soup left on the stove
I hear the last car leaving
Down the driveway and up the road
It's so sweet of Jim and Joan
To make a trip so long
I guess now I'll be making friends with gone.

The flowers they were beautiful
And everyone so kind
I thought how you'd have loved to see
so many dear friends at one time
After all the stories
and the toasts till nearly dawn
I guess now I'll be making friends with gone

I'm so glad we had those last days
laughing and crying and the jokes you made.
Like every time you drove away
you said I love you
We called out we love you too

Just a little longer now
I don't want to go to bed
Maybe just another walk
Down Cooper Road instead.
If anybody asks you just how I'm getting on
Tell them I'm still making friends with gone, now
Forever making friends with gone

Shari Ulrich composed this beautiful song and sang it at my mother Yetta's funeral, relating her experiences with the loss and grief following deaths involving close family and friends.

Losses in life are natural

In everyday life, we experience losses. As children, we experience loss when we go to kindergarten and leave our parents at home, or when a good friend is in a different class than we are or moves to a different school.

Loss is a normal experience of living

Losses can be tangible, like the death of a person or pet, or symbolic, like the loss of a dream. Some losses are clear, such as when a person dies suddenly—one day they are there and the next day they are not. Other losses are more ambiguous and difficult to identify, such as the loss of cognitive functioning with dementia.

Multiple losses occur with dying

Dying often involves multiple losses for the person and family

We experiences losses when someone important to us becomes very ill or dies. When an ill person cannot interact with us in their usual way, we both experience losses. This could mean the loss of a walking partner or a life partner. The point to remember is that the family and the ill person suffer losses when the person's abilities decline, mutual activities disappear, and the relationship changes.

It is sometimes possible to see a positive side to loss. For example, a family member might experience a more rewarding career when moving to a new job, and that will partially compensate for the loss resulting from no longer being near friends and community. The meaning of the loss to the person is what determines their response to the loss. Because each loss will have unique meaning for each person, based on their own life and experiences, it follows that each person will respond in their own way to loss.

Ambiguous losses are difficult

Ambiguous losses are those that are not clearly defined, for example, the many losses experienced by the family of a person with progressive dementia. The person is still alive but is not the same as they once were.

> When Mom could no longer care for herself and had to be placed in a facility, I had to be like the mother advocating for my "child." I still loved her, but it was different and my emotions were all mixed up. Sometimes I felt sad, but I was also angry and scared. I lost the mom I knew long before she died. But I couldn't really grieve the loss like I could have if she had died, because she was still alive. It was a difficult time and very few people understood what I was feeling.

Unexpected losses are difficult

Some losses are expected or "certain" while others are unexpected. In general, unexpected losses are more difficult to endure because the person cannot prepare for them mentally or emotionally. Therefore, by helping the dying person and their family prepare and plan for expected losses, PSWs can ease the process of declining health and dying by reducing the number of unexpected losses.

As a PSW, understanding the certainties of declining health and dying, as well as the nature of grief, will help guide your interactions with the person and their family.

To open conversations about the meaning of loss, you could ask questions like these:

> You have lived in your home for a long time on your own. How are you feeling about the move to assisted living?

I've noticed that it seems harder for you to get around without your walker late-ly. How is that for you?

I'm happy to prepare meals for you, but you have told me that you love to cook. How are you feeling about handing that off to someone else? Please let me know what your meal preferences are and I will do my best to accommodate them.

Multiple losses are difficult

It all began when Len woke up one day and his speech was slurred. The kids and I laughed at him. Then he began tripping over things and having trouble using his hands. By the time he was diagnosed with ALS, we stopped laughing. It seemed that every day he experienced one more loss. He became frustrated. Sometimes he yelled at me. Going for our daily walk, having a pleasant drive, playing cards, watching TV, entertaining our friends, all became impossible. All the things that gave our life meaning and happiness disappeared one by one. After a while he could do nothing for himself. Our relationship became that of patient and caregiver. Life as we had known it was gone forever. Some days I would lie on my bed and sob. One time I was interrupted in my crying by the sound of him crying in the other room. It just broke my heart. I realized then that grief begins long before a person dies.

People with life-threatening diseases experience multiple ongoing losses because of declining health. This may include the loss of the future that the dying person and their loved ones had hoped for, loss of activities and work they enjoyed, or loss of independence and control over much of their daily routine. Even when a person is familiar with loss, the intensity of their grief over a loss may surprise them.

People often struggle when losing their role in the family—for example, as the provider, as the parent, or as the partner. Many people struggle with losing their independence. When a person requires help to accomplish daily tasks, they may feel sad, frustrated, and angry because they can no longer do these things for them-selves. Some will fear becoming a burden.

When people experience repeated losses, one after another, they may feel that they are losing their quality of life. People often define themselves by what they do, so they may lose their sense of self when they can no longer participate in their daily activities.

Support people experiencing losses by listening, empathizing and communicating with the care team

PSWs can support people who are grieving multiple losses by listening to how the losses are affecting them and by remembering that each loss will have unique meaning for the person. What one person considers a major loss may be a minor loss to someone else. You can communicate the person's feeling about their losses to the care team so that the team can also provide support.

Understanding Grief

Grief is our response to loss

Grief is a normal response to loss. It is the natural, subjective, and complex reaction to a perceived loss. The word "grieve" comes from the Latin and Old French words meaning "heavy" and "burden," respectively. Grieving people frequently describe feeling weighed down or burdened.

Over 50 years ago, Elizabeth Kübler-Ross pioneered work on loss and grief by asking dying people and their loved ones what they were going through and what they needed from professionals. She was valuable in getting people talking about death, dying, loss, and grief, and proposed what she called the stages of grief. Kübler-Ross identified shock and disbelief, anger, bargaining, depression, and acceptance as the stages of grief people experience when they face their death. The stages seemed to resonate with many people, possibly because the stages made the variety of emotions of grief seem normal.

An incorrect understanding evolved, wherein grieving people were thought to move sequentially through each grief stage, resolving the emotions of each stage before proceeding. This was not Kübler-Ross's intent. People also mistakenly thought that the goal was for people to "accept" their illness and their death. We know now that many people do not want to accept death or the loss of a loved one. They do not want to "let go and move on."

Grief specialists no longer teach that people grieve in specific stages or that the goal of the grieving process is to accept the loss or find closure. While people who lose a loved one usually find ways to adapt to the loss and experience joy again, it is also true that grief often "walks with them" for the rest of their lives. This is an important perspective, because the goal shifts then to supporting people to find their way on their very personal and unique journey.

Colin Murray Parkes, a British psychiatrist and grief specialist, says that grief is the price we pay for love. If we ignore this truth, we will be unprepared to experience loss in our life or support other people in their grief.

Grief is a whole person experience

Grief is experienced and expressed in many different ways

When Lee's partner died, Lee was in shock for several months. His chest hurt, like his heart had actually broken. He didn't respond to his friends and family when they invited him out for a walk or to share a meal. He felt numb at times and then at other times would burst into tears without warning. He railed at a God that had always been a comforting source of strength. None of it made sense to him.

Grief is a whole person experience that affects every area of a grieving person's life. Human beings experience and express grief in many different ways.

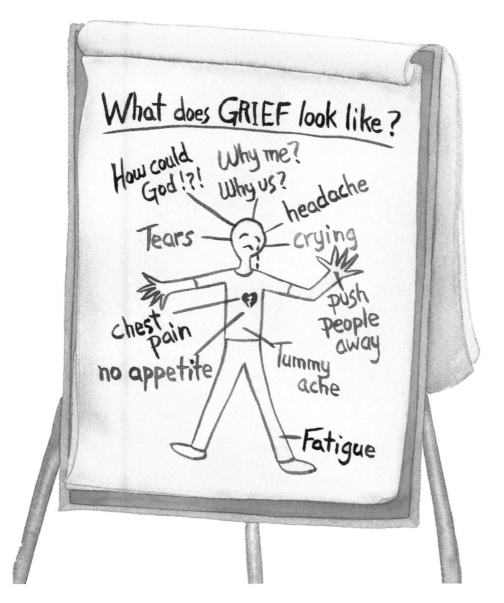

Physical

As in the story of Lee above, grief can be felt as an aching in the stomach, head, or chest, or as fatigue, restlessness, or listlessness. Sleeping can be difficult, even when the person is exhausted. Fatigue can be overwhelming. Some people have no appetite, while others take comfort in eating.

Social

Some grieving people find it impossible to be with friends and family because conversations that are not about grief seem trivial, yet if they do talk about their grief, they feel vulnerable and exposed. Others find that they need family and friends to distract them from their emotions and may feel frightened, lonely, and even resentful when family and friends leave. Still others worry that they will upset other people if they speak of their grief and so prefer to be silent.

Grief is the whole body response to loss

Emotional

The emotions of grief can feel overwhelming. Sadness is a common emotion of grief, as are anger, depression, irritability, annoyance, intolerance, and frustration. A person's feelings can be more intense with sleep deprivation, ongoing decline in functioning, the fear of being a burden, the fear of separation, and the challenges of facing the unknown. While some people readily express emotion through tears or angry outbursts, others may be more comfortable keeping their emotions to themselves.

Spiritual

It is common for people who are grieving to question their beliefs and long-held world views as they try to adjust to their new reality and find meaning in the loss and the situation. This may be particularly painful and surprising for those who have held strong beliefs and found comfort in those beliefs.

Mental

A grieving person may have difficulty thinking clearly. For some people, their mind is busy, going over and over the course of events, trying to recall or understand what happened. Others have trouble concentrating and may be forgetful, have difficulty doing things that were easy, or have difficulty learning new things. The person may become easily confused and feel mentally exhausted even after sleeping, or may forget simple things, such as how to get to the store or how to cook a basic meal. Some people fear they are going crazy.

In your caregiving, you will care for people who grieve in a variety of ways.

People who like to draw or reflect may find using a body map helpful to understand their "whole person" experience of grief.

Several factors influence a person's grief

A person's grieving is as unique as the person and their experiences

The intensity of a person's grief is influenced by the timing of the loss, the nature of the loss, what the loss means in terms of the progression of their illness, and how the loss affects their ability to maintain hope. A dying person's perception of a loss and its effect on quality of life are the most significant influences on their grief. Consider these losses:

- The loss of independent living when moving into an assisted living facility
- The loss of independence when help is required for daily activities
- The loss of privacy when a person needs total care

While these losses are common as illness progresses, the meaning of the loss will be different for each person. For example, while one person may grieve the loss of the ability or opportunity to cook, another may be relieved that someone else is now responsible for doing the grocery shopping and making meals. Understanding the meaning of the loss to the person at the time will be important to understanding their grief.

People experience grief differently over time

One of the truths about grief is that grief does not end. The intensity and energy of grief usually decrease over time, but in some form grief is woven into the fabric of a person's life.

Grief changes

Initially I was completely wiped out. I dragged myself through each day. I could not think clearly to make decisions. I had to rely on others to help me sort out the big stuff. I was unable to eat. The first year after my husband died in the accident, I was a mess.

People were kind. They brought meals. They drove the kids to school. They put snow tires on the car. They winterized the house. I don't know where I was, but I know I did not function well.

Now, the kids and I are managing better. We still miss him. I think of him every day. I miss him especially at special times for the kids. But, it does not hurt so much anymore. And I don't cry as much as I used to cry. It is easier. The blanket of grief is not as heavy. There are holes in it, and it is more a part of my life.

People grieve in different and unique ways

Greta and Jack cared for their adult son for months when he was dying. Greta attended to his every need. After his death her days seemed endless and her grief was overwhelming. She sobbed for hours at a time. She talked with others who understood and who allowed her to cry.

Support grieving people by listening and empathizing

Jack was dry eyed. He arranged the funeral, found hotels for out of town relatives who came to the funeral, gave a brilliant eulogy, and later made a bench with a plaque dedicated to his son. He applied to the city to design and build a small memorial garden in a local park where the bench would be placed.

Two researchers, Kenneth J. Doka and Terry L. Martin, created the terms "intuitive griever" and "instrumental griever" to help us understand two styles of grieving.[2] An intuitive griever is expressive and freely shows their emotions. This grieving style has traditionally been associated with women but is *not* limited to women. An instrumental griever is active in their grief. They express themselves by taking concrete or practical steps. This style of grief is traditionally associated with men but is *not* limited to men.

Instrumental and Intuitive Grievers

---

2 T. Martin, and K. Doka, *Men Don't Cry … Women Do: Transcending Gender Stereotypes of Grief* (New York: Brunner Mazel/Taylor & Francis, 2000).

The story of Greta and Jack shows her to be an intuitive griever. Greta's emotions are easily accessible. In her grief, she cries frequently and sometimes feels like she lacks control. She finds support in being with other people. At times, the intensity of her feelings is frightening to her and she is often fatigued. Her focus is on her feelings, not on accomplishing tasks.

Jack is an instrumental griever. He stays busy attending to tasks, focuses on caring for others, and appears to be coping with daily activities. He makes meaning of his son's death by memorializing him and preparing a park bench to celebrate his life. Jack struggles to maintain control while he feels deep pain, turmoil, and anxiety. He copes with the loss in the same manner that he copes with other problems that he needs to solve. He appreciates privacy. He does not welcome questions that address feelings but may accept help with his projects.

The way a person grieves is neither right nor wrong. It simply is.

Greta and Jack grieve in different ways. Both Greta and Jack are adapting to the world without their son. Neither way is right or wrong. The two stories above illustrate different grieving styles. Knowing a person's grieving style makes it less likely that you will judge, evaluate, or label their behaviour. Knowing their grieving style makes is easier to support them in their grieving.

For example, Greta might appreciate attending a support group as she grieves, while Jack might prefer to work with the community to establish the memorial garden.

Caregivers need to refrain from judging or labelling the behaviour of grieving people. Instead, you can support them by letting them know that their grief and ways of expressing grief are normal, and by helping them identify their own strengths in coping and accept the way others are grieving. When you give people the chance to identify what is helpful to them, you can better support them.

People may use denial to cope with overwhelming loss and grief

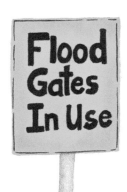

Every person has a unique response to bad news, grief, and loss. While some people ask questions, take notes, and read as much as they can to understand what is happening, others appear to withdraw and reject the information and its implications. When a person appears to ignore the reality of a diagnosis, prognosis, or suggestion (e.g., that they need to use a walker), they may be labelled as "in denial." In some cultures, being in denial is judged as a weakness that needs fixing. Caregivers need to understand that denial is a valid coping mechanism for people managing difficult or frightening information that may lead to feelings of overwhelming loss and grief.

It may be helpful to consider that people use denial as a way to reduce the flow of bad news, allowing only as much information in as they can comfortably tolerate. This situation is not unlike that of the farmer who builds a floodgate to manage the flow of water onto his land. The floodgate limits the amount of water coming in and preserves the land. In this analogy, the water is the flow of bad news and closing the floodgate (denial) is the person's way to limit the flow of information. Each person has a unique capacity to process information, and some people create an internal floodgate to control the flow of bad news as a means of self-preservation. Denial is one method people use to control the flow of difficult information so that they can deal with it in smaller amounts. It is another way of saying, "I'm just not ready for that information yet. I need more time to take it all in."

It's important to remember that each person will respond differently to bad news and will absorb the information as they are able. You can acknowledge to the person and their family that it is normal for people to take in information at different rates. This may help family members be less judgemental with each other.

Denial may be a coping strategy

You may support the person by saying something like this:

> Sometimes it takes people a bit of time to adapt to all this information. That is all right.

Supporting a Grieving Person

Supportive strategies include inviting the person to talk, listening attentively to what they say, and responding with compassion and acceptance. It is important to remember that each person is unique, so support will be different for each person. Below are some strategies PSWs can try when supporting someone dealing with losses and grief.

Acknowledging

It may be helpful to acknowledge the loss, grief, and mixed emotions the person is experiencing.

> You have had many changes in the last few months. How has that been for you?

> This seems really hard for you. I hear the pain in your voice.

Mixed emotions are common in people who experience losses. Family members feel sadness about the impending loss of a loved one and at the same time may also feel guilty for being well, for wanting time for themselves, or for being frustrated and angry at having to take time away from work to be a caregiver. The dying person may feel grateful that you prepare the meals and help with personal care and at the same time resent that they need your help. And, after death occurs, a family member may express both relief and grief, especially if there have been many losses to deal with during a long and slow dying process. These are all examples of mixed emotions and a range of emotions. There are no good or bad emotions in the grieving process, just as there is no right or wrong way to grieve. It may be helpful to acknowledge that emotions, like relationships, are complicated. You can support a person who is expressing mixed emotions by acknowledging for them that relationships are complicated, that both caregiving and being sick are difficult, and that having mixed feelings is normal.

Acknowledge

Empathizing and reflecting

Empathy is the ability to understand how the other person is feeling and includes being willing to get close to another person's emotional pain without needing to hide it or fix it. Sometimes it can be helpful to reflect back what the person has said or what you have observed. Consider how you might use phrases like the following, remembering that to be credible you must use your own words.

Empathize

> *It sounds like you are having a tough day. Is there anything I can do to help?*
>
> *It seems like your feelings of sorrow are overwhelming.*
>
> *It sounds like you are really struggling to try to find meaning in what is happening to you [your loved one].*
>
> *These are big questions that you are asking. Do you want to talk about them, or are you happy to just think about them?*

Leaving room for silence

It takes courage and confidence to be able to witness deep grief and stay present, perhaps only offering a gentle touch or companioning in silence. Silence can be a sign that the person feels comfortable in your company. Sometimes the mere presence of another human can be comforting. Silence, however, can be awkward if the other person feels responsible for entertaining or engaging with you. It can be difficult to decide whether silence is welcome or not. It may be difficult for you to keep silent if you are accustomed to talking or feel it is your responsibility to keep the conversation going.

Be silent

Many people associate silence with emptiness or just an absence of conversation. In fact, silence is full of presence; there is always something going on in the spaces between our words and actions. Embracing silence clears space for whatever needs to happen. When working with people who are profoundly ill, grieving, overwhelmed by change and loss, or anxious and fearful about what lies ahead, silence can be a gift that allows the person the time and space to collect their thoughts, to reflect on the immensity of death, or to consider questions like "Why me?" that have no answers. Being comfortable with silence requires an ability to trust yourself and the person you are with, in order to give up control of the space that silence creates.

If conversation meets the needs of the person receiving care, then talking is appropriate. It's a good idea to check regularly to see if the person is tired of talking. A conversation can be a useful distraction from discomfort, but it can also be exhausting. If you are not sure whether someone wants you to continue to talk, you might say something like, "I don't want to tire you out with conversation. I can just sit here with you quietly if you would prefer."

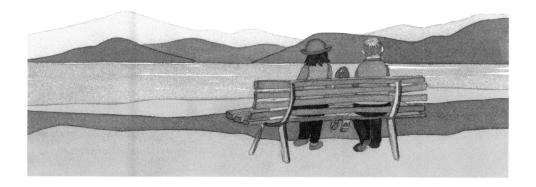

> Perhaps the most important thing we bring to another person is the silence in us, not the sort of silence that is filled with unspoken criticism or hard withdrawal. The sort of silence that is a place of refuge, of rest, of acceptance of someone as they are. We are all hungry for this other silence. It is hard to find. In its presence we can remember something beyond the moment, a strength on which to build a life. Silence is a place of great power and healing.
> —*Rachel Naomi Remen*[3]

Individualizing care

It is important for caregivers to remember to allow the grieving person to guide the care. You can be curious and focus on the person, and invite the person to describe what is helpful, what they appreciate people doing to help them. You know too that family members will grieve and will express their grief in different ways. Your compassionate response to each person will model that there are many normal ways to express grief and many ways to support a person in their grief.

You might say,

> *In every family or social group there will be people who express their grief in different ways.*

> *What you are telling me is completely normal.*

Reflecting on people's grieving style will help you understand how to support them. Instrumental grievers may respond best to concrete information about grief. They may benefit from having projects and assignments to address the needs of the people involved. Intuitive grievers may find it most helpful when people listen to them and allow them to explore and express feelings. Groups such as a breast cancer support group and the Family Caregivers' Network Society[4] may meet the person's need for sharing.

Individualize

---

3 N.R. Remen, *Kitchen Table Wisdom: Stories That Heal* (New York: Putnam, 1997).

4 Family Caregivers' Network Society, http://www.fcns-caregiving.org.

When Robert's wife died, people from the church and others that he barely knew in his neighbourhood left many casseroles and baked goods on his doorstep. He had no appetite and felt guilty when the food went bad.

Regina was the PSW caring for Robert. She wondered why Robert didn't eat the food and why he was not expressing gratitude for the meals. She resisted the urge to judge him and decided to be curious. One day she asked him, "Robert, of all the things that you have to deal with right now, what would you say is the most difficult for you?"

He looked her in the eye and said, "I just miss her. I feel so awfully lonely I just want to lie down and die."

Regina's heart felt like it was melting. She put her hand on his shoulder and sat down beside him. "What do you need the most right now?"

She was very surprised when he said, "I want some company. I don't want the casseroles, I want someone to sit down and share a cup of tea with me." Regina and Robert then talked about how he could make that happen.

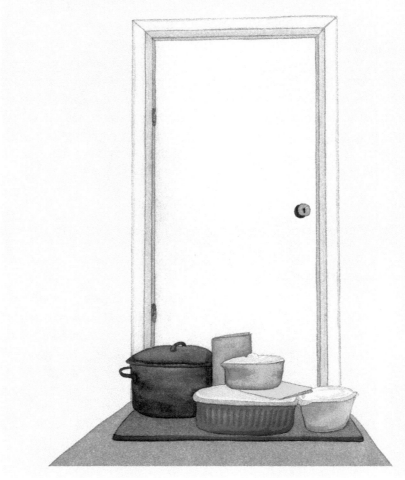

People who are more intuitive grievers, or "feelers," may appreciate being offered the opportunity to express their grief and conversations about their experience.

Do you want to talk about how this is for you?

As a PSW, you can help in the following ways:

- Remind the person that it takes time to grieve but that they will adjust with time.

    It is normal for this to take a while. Do not feel that you have to rush to recover or to adapt. It is normal for people to have a lot of emotion.

- Support the person if they struggle to think clearly or feel disorganized or disoriented.

    It is hard when you are not able to think as clearly as you normally do. Would it be helpful to write notes about these concerns so that you can remember to talk about them with the doctor [your kids]?

    It is common for people to feel disoriented and mixed up. Would it be helpful if we reviewed the calendar again?

- Support the person to meet their commitments and handle problems that arise.

    You mentioned that your kids are coming today and want to meet with the community nurse. Can you tell the nurse what time your kids will be here?

- Support the person to link with community resources.

    I think your dad might like the recreation activities. Do you want to connect with the activity person?

People who are more instrumental, action-oriented grievers may attend planned activities but may seek private ways to express feelings, such as listening to a sad song or watching a video alone.

You mention feeling isolated in your role as a caregiver. I understand that there is an online support group for family caregivers. They meet each week, and all you need is a phone to connect. They provide information and education about family caregiving. Do you want me to get you that information?

Would you like to watch one of your favourite old-time movies that you save for special occasions? I wonder if one of those emotional movies might be a nice way to think about your own feelings in a private way.

Making room for tears

Crying is a normal, healthy response to grief. Sometimes people try to stop people from crying by handing them tissues, patting them on the back and saying "shhh," distracting them, or putting a positive spin on the person's grief. Silence and gently acknowledging that "It's so hard right now" may make space for tears. Sometimes other people's tears will trigger your own. This is normal and can be very comforting to the other person because they can see that you understand. As long as the focus stays on the person you are with and does not move to you, it is okay to shed a few tears. (You may want to discuss your emotions later with a colleague or supervisor.)

Identifying people who need extra support

Some people need additional support when grieving after the death of a loved one. In some cases, this is because the death was sudden, difficult, or complicated by other challenging life events. In other cases, people's grief may be intensified by personal factors, for example, being socially isolated, being the primary caregiver for a long time, having pre-existing challenges with the person who died, having mental or physical health issues themselves, or being in the midst of a personal, unrelated crisis.

Ask yourself whether this person might benefit from additional support

Social factors that may affect bereavement are a lack of financial resources, difficult family dynamics, or lifestyle changes resulting from illness and death. Examples of these challenges include the isolation entailed in long-term caregiving, needing to relocate, loss of a job, or changes in the bereaved person's ability to live independently.

As a PSW, you may see or hear from the bereaved person, other family members, friends, or colleagues that the bereaved person is struggling. While it is completely normal to lose one's appetite or not feel like getting dressed, it is a concern if the normal signs of grief seem exaggerated and/or occur over an extended time. You may notice that the person is not coping well if they show consistent and debilitating fatigue or an inability to take care of daily business, talk about self-harm, or express an ongoing sense of purposelessness.

You can make a big difference in a person's life by showing, through your words and actions, that you support them and care about them.

When circumstances of the death or social or personal factors have made grieving especially difficult, and when the grieving person appears to need extra support, it is important that you record this information and report it to the nurse.

Remembering

Emotional pains cannot be fixed with "emotional morphine."

The physical pains and discomfort discussed in Chapter 4 can often be decreased through the use of medications and comfort measures. However, when a person is dying, there are psychosocial pains that cannot be fixed. There is no "emotional morphine" that can ease deep suffering. The other reality is that not only can you not fix deep suffering, but it is not your job to try to fix. It is your job to provide support. Chapter 3 contains more information about this topic.

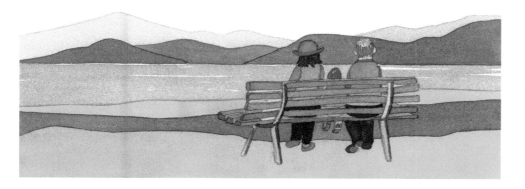

For additional information on supporting children whose loved one is dying, refer to Appendix B.

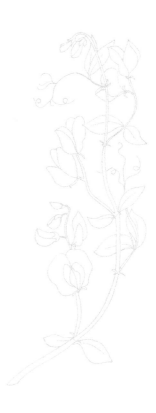

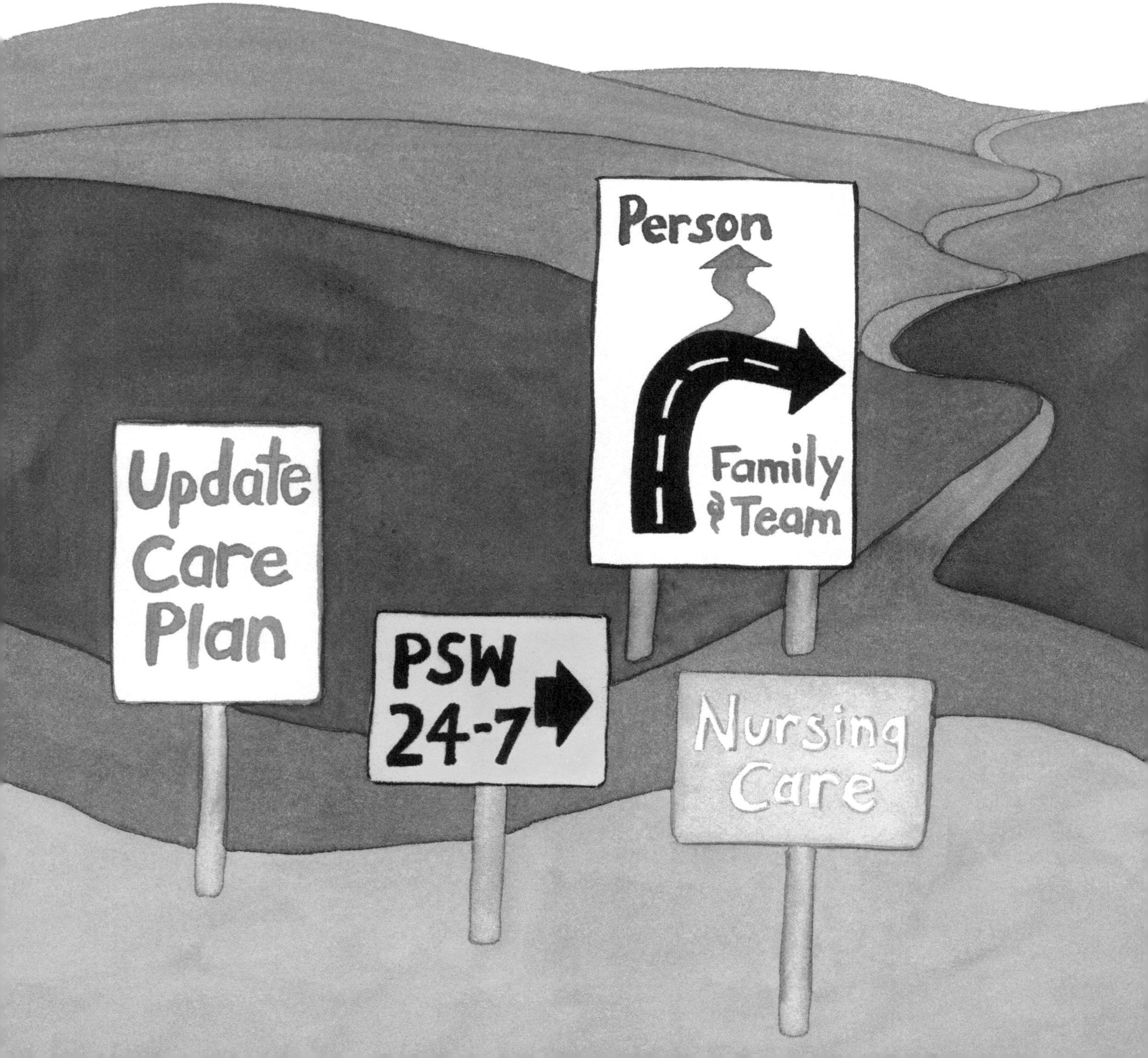
Person
Family & Team
Update Care Plan
PSW 24-7
Nursing Care

6

Caring in the Last Days and Hours

Chapter 1 of *Integrating a Palliative Approach: Essentials for Personal Support Workers* is about preparing yourself to provide care. In Chapter 2, four common patterns, or trajectories, of dying and some of the challenges associated with each of those patterns are described. Chapter 3 is about the principles of hospice palliative care (HPC) and the concept of integrating a palliative approach into care as a way to address the needs of the dying person and their family. Chapter 4 discusses a few tools to help you provide excellent physical care, describes the common symptoms that dying people experience, identifies questions that you can adapt to help you gather information to use in assessing how best to care, and provides information about many measures you can use to provide comfort to dying people. Psycho-social issues and strategies for providing support are discussed in Chapter 5.

This chapter is the last in this book that discusses care of the dying person and their family, specifically in the last days and hours of the person's life. The focus in this chapter is on preparing the family to provide care (depending on their ability and willingness to do so), the physical changes that occur in the dying person, ways to support the person and their family, and care of the body after death and care of the family. What to do when death is sudden, and the emerging home funeral movement, are also discussed briefly.

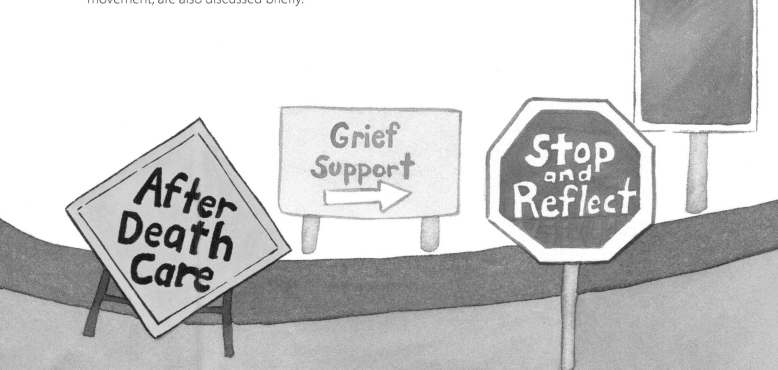

As you can imagine, the last days and hours can be a special time, a sad time, and a sacred time for the dying person and their family. This time can also be challenging. You can help by providing a calm and empathetic presence. Calmness can be contagious, and your presence can help reduce anxiety and stress. Your presence, your way of being with the person and family, your offer of kind, supportive care may be remembered for years.

It is important that you prepare to adapt what you do as needs change, and that you provide the support that is needed in the moment. When the family arrives after the person has died, you may need to step back so the family can be right at the bedside. You may need to sit at the bedside because the family wants to meet in another room. Being aware of your beliefs and baggage will help you put your preferences aside and focus on the needs of those for whom you care.

In the words of Stephen Levine, an author and teacher well known for his work on death and dying, "Working with people in crisis is similar to reading Braille—you need to feel your way moment by moment." Remember those words!

Preparing to Care

The health care team can help prepare the family (and staff) to care for the person in the last days and hours by doing the following:
- Sharing information
- Responding to questions
- Arranging for support and resources
- Developing a plan for the time of death
- Identifying rituals and preferences for care following death

Sharing Information

Families need information to understand what is happening

Families report that information is one of the things they need the most when their loved one is dying. Information can help families understand what is happening and what to expect, when death might occur, what they can do to be supportive, and whom they need to call if they have concerns or if needs arise.

The Canadian Hospice Palliative Care Association (CHPCA) identifies the components of the process of providing care as follows: assessment, information sharing, decision making, care planning, care implementation, and confirmation (evaluation). Sharing information with family about common physical changes in the dying person in the last days and hours is one of the most important things the team can do.

If the family asks questions such as "What changes can I expect in the last days and hours?" as a PSW you support information sharing when you

- Acknowledge and validate the family's questions
- Connect the family with the nurse, or a counsellor or social worker, who can answer their questions
- Share agency or facility educational brochures about what to expect as death nears, which the family can review while waiting to meet with the nurse
- Ensure that the family knows how to access the team
- Remember that as you provide care you are modelling comfort measures for the family

Acknowledge family's concerns and connect with the health care team

Depending on where you work, your expertise in information sharing, and your relationship with the person and family, the nurse may assist you in sharing information.

Responding to Questions

Families often ask (or wonder) how much longer their loved one will live and what they can expect in the last days and hours. Responding to such questions with "I am only a PSW, I don't know" is both unhelpful and inappropriate. As a PSW, remember that you are an important member of the team. You are not responsible for answering such questions, but you are responsible for responding to them in a way that is helpful. Below are some suggestions that will help you acknowledge and validate the family's questions, consider the family's needs, and explore what the family understands about the timing of death.

"That's a valid question to ask"

When the family asks a question like "How much longer does he have to live?" you can acknowledge and validate their question by saying,

> That is a question we are often asked. It is not an easy question to ask, and it is not an easy question to answer.

The family might ask such a question for many reasons; for example; they may need to arrange for people from out of town to visit, or decide how to balance work with being at the bedside. You can explore with the family whether they have any specific reasons for asking the question.

> It would help me and the care team to understand a bit more about what this question means to you. Is there a specific reason you are asking this question now? If we can better understand your needs, then we can better help you.

"If we can better understand your needs, then we will be more able to help you"

Understanding the meaning behind the question will help the nurse or physician provide the needed information and support.

It is helpful to find out if family members have their own sense of how long the dying person will live. You might consider asking,

"What are your thoughts on what is happening?"

I'm wondering if you have any sense of timing yourself? For example, have you noticed any changes in your father's condition lately? And if so, do you have a sense of what they might mean?

Asking this question can be very helpful. The family may have a much better idea than the care team. They may know something about the person's goals or personality that may affect the time of death. For example, the family may respond with answers like these:

I think she is waiting for her grandchild to be born.

She always does everything very carefully and never rushes at anything, so I think she might linger for a while.

On the other hand, the family may have no idea when their loved one will die and may need help to adjust to the immediacy of death. For example, I remember a dying woman who wanted me to be with her when she shared some advice with her teenage daughter. After we had that very intimate time together, and when I was alone with the daughter, I asked her if she had a sense of how long her mom might live.

The daughter replied, "I used to think that she had a long time, but now I don't think she has very long … maybe six months."

I was concerned when I heard this, as I figured that the mom had only days to live. I talked with the daughter and suggested that I did not think it would be that long, and that I thought it would be a good idea for her to talk with the counsellor and the doctor later that day. I was able to arrange some supports for her.

PSWs can acknowledge questions, clarify needs and explore perceptions of family

Once you have acknowledged the question, clarified why the person is asking it, and found out how long the family thinks the person may live, you will need to share this question and information with the nurse or other health care professional. You might say to the family,

I would like to talk with the nurse about your question, your thoughts, and your needs. I will ask the nurse to speak with you and share thoughts on your father's prognosis.

In your role as a PSW, it is appropriate for you to acknowledge the question, clarify needs, and explore the family's understanding.

Arranging for Support and Resources

In the same sense that "it takes a village to raise a child," my mother, Yetta, repeatedly said, "and it takes a village to care for the dying." This is particularly true for people dying at home. When there are only a few caregivers in the home, providing care for a person dying there becomes challenging. Often the additional support from PSWs makes a person's desire to die at home a possibility.

The introductory section of this chapter mentioned physical changes that occur when death is imminent. Family and inexperienced caregivers might not view these changes as normal or expected. When the changes occur, the family may need someone to call, to talk with about the changes, to provide a visit or phone support. Therefore, one key ingredient in helping people remain at home through to death is the availability of support day and night, seven days a week.

You will benefit from knowing what care the health care team provides and how the team provides it in the community or care setting where you work. Knowing how and when to ask for help can make the difference between preventing a crisis and having to transfer a dying person to a hospital in the last days. Prepare yourself to respond to the family's questions, such as those below, whether you are working in a care facility or providing support in the home.

Whom do I call if I have questions or concerns?

Who is available at night and on weekends to respond to my needs and questions?

How do I get help if my loved one is uncomfortable in the night?

What do I do in the middle of the night if his pain gets worse?

How can I get more hours of PSW care?

What other resources are available to us for providing care in the home?

Prepare to respond to these common questions, even if the response is, "That's a good question, let's ask the nurse."

In some communities, the health care team is not available at night or on the weekends. Where that is the case, it is important for the health care team to strengthen the informal caregivers, including friends, relatives, and neighbours. In the Yukon, the HPC team from Whitehorse provides education sessions in remote areas to prepare the "village" to care. In other remote communities, the family caregivers are provided with an emergency contact number they can phone day or night, seven days a week.

It is especially important to help family members who are providing care in the home setting understand how to access available resources, but it is equally important in acute care or long-term care facilities to have resources and know how to access them.

Developing a Plan for the Time of Death

When I was pregnant with my first child, I was keen to develop a birth care plan. I wanted to be sure that the care team knew what I wanted and would respond to the needs that arose during the birthing process as discussed in our prior conversations and noted in my care plan.

And so it is with dying. When the time comes, I want my caregivers to know what is important to me! I want my caregivers to know my hopes and preferences for my dying and the care of my body after I die. And I expect that, just as my birthing plan was adjusted to meet my and my baby's needs during the birthing process, my family and care team will honour my preferences when I am dying and will adjust to meet needs as they arise. Whether I die at home or in a hospital, hospice, or long-term care setting, the essence of who I am, what I am, and what I hope for can be honoured.

As death approaches, the more hypothetical discussions that may have occurred years and months before, and the care plans that were developed weeks or days ago, can now be fine-tuned to meet the needs when dying occurs.

A care plan needs to address the physical changes and psychosocial implications of the changes that occur in the last days and hours. See page 160 for more information on the expected changes and ways to support both the dying person and the family.

In developing a care plan, it is important for family and staff to know what to do when death occurs. You and they will need to know the following:
- Whether there is a signed Do Not Resuscitate (DNR) form and where is it located
- Who will "pronounce" the death

The person who pronounces the death confirms that the person has died by checking that their heart is not beating, the person is not breathing, and their pupils are fixed and dilated. In some provinces, the family is allowed to pronounce death if the physician has previously signed an "Expected Death at Home" form. This form indicates that the doctor or nurse will not be attending the death. The form directs the family when to contact the funeral home following death.

In addition to knowing what to do when death occurs, it is helpful to know the following:
- Who notifies the physician or nurse to pronounce death
- What to do if the physician or nurse who is supposed to pronounce the death is not available
- Who needs to be notified following death

As a PSW, you need to be aware of any preferences the dying person or their family has expressed with regard to specific rituals and traditions that they would like to be observed after the person's death, and how they want the body to be cared for.

Identifying Rituals and Preferences for Care Following Death

Below are some questions that may help PSWs open the door to conversations with the family as they consider what they want and need at the time of their loved one's death and following death.

The time following death can be a special and a sacred time. Is there anything special you want to do or have happen when death occurs or following death?

Are there any traditions important in your family, culture, or religious community that you would like to observe?

Is there someone in your extended family that you want to talk with in case there are traditions of which you are not aware?

Are there any requirements or preferences that relate to not touching the body following death?

Is there someone you want to be here with you when death occurs or following death?

Is there something that you think the dying person would like or not like done?

Some people like to have the person's body removed soon after death. Others want the body to remain in the home for a time. Have you thought about this?

What might be helpful to you as a family, or as caregivers, following death?

> Use these door openers to conversations about rituals and preferences around dying and after death

It is important to record and report any specific rituals that will affect how and when care is provided, and anything else that will require special considerations from the health care team. Communicating any special requests to the health care team is also advised.

> Record and report any specific rituals or instructions that will affect care surrounding dying

Questions like those below may help you consider the needs of the family:

Who do you want present at the time of death or following death?

Who do you want to notify that death has occurred?

Is there anyone you would like me to notify?

It there a spiritual leader or support person you would like us to contact?

In addition to considering how to care for the body and support the family, it is important to know whether a funeral home will be involved and, if so, its contact information. The family may want to keep the body in the home for a period of time following death. For some families, this is a matter of hours, but others will want the body to stay in the home until the time for burial. Throughout the world, people have many different traditions and preferences that relate to death. If the family is concerned that they may not be able to act in accordance with the rituals and

> Record any preferences for care of the body after death

traditions that they want to observe, you can connect them with the appropriate person on the health care team who can provide information and support.

Providing Compassion: It's Hard to Be Family

People who are involved in palliative care often say, "Caring for the dying person is easy. It is caring for the family that is difficult."

Families need compassion, not judgement

Of course it is easier, or simpler, to care for an unresponsive person than to care for a group of people who have come together to be with, care for, and make decisions for a family member who is dying. Just imagine all that is happening for this group of people! Imagine each person and what that person might be experiencing. Imagine what the whole person experience of grief might be like for each person involved—the emotions, the struggle to think, the stress and pains in their body, the spiritual angst, the difficulty relating to other people. All these things are normal. Now think of these people who have come together as a group, perhaps as a family, with who knows what history of relationships, styles, personalities, struggles, wounds, communication blocks—imagine that they are together, perhaps for the first time in years, perhaps because they are drawn to close what have been difficult relationships, perhaps dancing a dance that they have danced for decades. Imagine that they are having to walk side by side with someone whose style does not mesh with theirs and whose presence irritates or reminds them of hard days gone by. Just imagine! You say that caring for the dying person is easier. Of course it is!

Let me share a few secrets with you.

Family need you to:
- empathize
- support
- acknowledge
- inform
- encourage

Caring for, or companioning, a loved one through to death can be a sacred and special experience, but it can also be a difficult and challenging one. Some family caregivers choose to take on that role, and others may feel that they had no choice and feel resentment for having to do so. Some people respond to the dying of a loved one by wanting to help, while others may find it too uncomfortable or frightening to be involved at all. It is normal for old, unresolved issues and feelings to bubble up to the surface when someone is dying, making family dynamics complex and sometimes even hard to watch. At other times, family members may actually be brought closer to one another by an impending death and the need to work together to make decisions and carry out a loved one's wishes.

The point is that people respond to a family member dying in all kinds of different ways, and this is normal and to be expected. It is also true that the ways in which people respond when a loved one is dying are strongly related to their history as a family, including the nature of their relationships with each other, and the physical and emotional distance that separates them, as well as their existing obligations to work and so on.

Family members need your understanding, your compassion, and your warmth. They do not need you to take sides, judge, or share your personal opinions. Be kind. They need you to empathize, support, acknowledge, inform, and encourage. I repeat: Be kind!

You would do well to remember the following:

- The dying person and the family are the unit of care. While you work to create a safe place for the person to die, try to create a safe place for the family too.
- Stress and grief may be a family's constant companions. Understand and accept the wide range of emotional responses that various family members experience.
- Respond to questions and concerns, even if it is simply to reply, "That is a good question. Can I connect you with the nurse who can discuss that in further detail?"

Strategies for supporting family with compassion

- Accurate information given in a timely way allows family members to anticipate changes, validate what they see, and participate in caregiving. It can also reduce fears and prevent unnecessary crises.
- Receiving conflicting messages from various members of the team is difficult for the person and the family. If a family is struggling with conflicting messages, talk with the nurse. When you share information with the family, make sure it is accurate and consistent with information the team provides and with the care plan.

Family caregivers may struggle with what professionals see as natural and normal changes in the dying process, because for many people these physical changes are not, in fact, normal in their experience of living! It may be difficult for them to understand and accept information that is new or challenges their personal experience or beliefs. Therefore, individual team members need to be willing to repeat information, perhaps in different ways. In this process, however, the consistency of the core information is crucial.

Physical Changes and Psychosocial Implications

Dying people experience some or all of these changes, in their own unique order and timing

Physical changes often occur during the last days and hours when a person is actively dying. Not all dying people experience every change, nor do they experience the changes in the order listed below. Anticipating the changes will validate what the family is seeing and will help the family participate in providing care.

It is helpful if you, as a PSW, understand the physical changes the dying person undergoes, as well as the emotional consequences for the family.

The following sections about these common changes during the last days and hours suggest ways that, together with those discussed in Chapter 4, will help you support the person and their family.

Common Physical Changes during the Last Days and Hours

Decreased physical strength and increased drowsiness

Reduced intake and difficulty swallowing

Delirium or confusion

Agitation and/or restlessness

Unresponsiveness

Irregular breathing

Congested breathing

Changes in skin colour and temperature

Muscle twitching

Dry eyes

Lack of urinary output and/or bowel and bladder incontinence

Decreased Physical Strength and Increased Drowsiness

As death nears, the dying person's strength decreases and the time spent sleeping increases, until eventually the person is sleeping most of the day. These are natural changes in the dying process.

Supporting the dying person

You can adapt the care plan to meet the needs and changing priorities of the person. For example, sleeping may be more important than a daily bed bath; visiting with family may be more important than visiting with friends. Keeping the care team informed of the changing needs and priorities is very important.

Adjust caregiving as needed

Supporting the family

The increased sleeping of the dying person can be difficult for their family, who may feel they are missing time with their loved one. Caregivers have heard family members say things such as "I knew she was dying in a few weeks, but I did not realize she would be sleeping most of that time." You can help in the following ways:

- Acknowledge that it is common for people to sleep more as death nears. You might say,

  It is normal for a dying person to sleep more and more as time passes.

- If the family expresses concerns that medication may be causing their loved one's drowsiness, encourage them to talk with the nurse or physician.
- Share information:
  - If the person's wakefulness follows a pattern, let the family know what times would provide ideal opportunities for visiting.
  - Explain that even enjoyable visits can be exhausting for the person, and discuss ways to limit visitors or the length of visits, and the possibility of restricting visits to immediate family.

Inform family that increased sleeping is normal

- Help the family find ways of being with their loved one whose energy is low. Depending on the interests of the person, this could include playing their favourite music, reading a special book, or reminiscing about good times.
- Let the family know that physical contact is important as people die. Even if a person is too weak to respond, they may find it reassuring to have physical contact, such as holding hands.
- Encourage family members to continue talking with the dying person and one another, because hearing familiar voices may comfort the person. The person's hearing might be the last sense to go.

Reduced Intake and Difficult Swallowing

Decreased intake is expected in last days and hours

In the last days and hours, a person's intake naturally decreases and changes from mixed fluids to clear fluids, from a mouthful to sips of fluids, and from sips to nothing by mouth. The person may begin having difficulty swallowing, followed by forgetting how to swallow and then becoming unable to swallow.

Supporting the dying person

As a PSW, you can help the dying person in these ways:
- Give the person thickened fluids if directed by the nurse or dietitian.
- Remind the person to swallow if they forget.
- Do not give anything by mouth if the person is coughing or choking on fluids.

Supporting the family

Encourage family to ask questions of health care team

The dying person's transition from eating and drinking to no longer eating or drinking can be particularly difficult and emotional for their family. As a PSW, you can support the family by doing the following:
- Acknowledge that this change is normal when a person is dying. Inform the family that even though it is a normal and expected change, it can also be a very difficult one to witness. Family members struggle with this transition, finding it hard to imagine that their loved one can no longer eat or drink and possibly understanding for the first time that the person is dying.
- Encourage the family to talk to or ask questions of the nurse, physician, or dietitian when they have concerns about the effects of decreased intake on their loved one and what the experience may be like for that person.

Good mouth care provides comfort when intake decreases

- Share information:
  - Inform the family of changes in the person's intake and ability to swallow.
  - Use family-friendly language. You might say,

    She is only taking sips of water.

    She is no longer able to swallow, but seems comforted when I freshen her mouth.

  - Explain the benefits of good mouth care and demonstrate how to give it if the family wants to participate in providing comfort measures.

Involving family in providing mouth care may comfort the person and family

  - Explore other ways to nurture, by asking questions. You might ask,

    Were there any activities that your mom liked that you might do now, like playing music, singing, sharing stories, giving her a gentle massage?

Delirium or Confusion

It is common for dying people to have periods of delirium in the last few days of life. The delirium may include confusion, misperceptions, and difficulties with focusing and separating events of the past, present, or future. If the person is very sleepy, the delirium may be less noticeable. If the person is awake, restless, and agitated, medications may help settle the person.

Supporting the dying person

These are some comfort measures to support the person who has delirium:

- Promptly report early signs of delirium to the nurse.
- Reorient and provide reassurance if the person is afraid or paranoid. You may say,

  Can you tell me what is happening? I don't see what you are seeing but I know that you do. You are safe. I am here with you and I have contacted the nurse.

- Allow the person to be in their delirium without reorientation if they appear to be comfortable.
- Offer soothing comfort measures such as warm blankets, massage, or healing touch.

A person who is calm in their delirium may not need to be reoriented

Dying people may see deceased loved ones or other entities during delirium or in the last days and hours. In HPC, this is referred to as "nearing death awareness," as defined by Maggie Callanan and Patricia Kelley in their classic book *Final Gifts: Understanding the Special Awareness, Needs, and Communications of the Dying.*[1] Many members of the health care team do not consider such behaviour to be a manifestation of delirium.

It may be appropriate for you to explore with the person what they are seeing. You might say,

"Tell me what you see"

  Tell me, what do you see?

  Tell me more about what you are experiencing.

Final Gifts

Maggie Callanan and Patricia Kelley, two hospice nurses, wrote about "nearing death awareness." They found that many dying people have visions of people who have already died. The authors relate how common it is for dying people to use metaphorical language and to experience restlessness and agitation as they talk about what they need in order to have a peaceful death. Callanan and Kelley suggest that rather than trying to point out reality to the dying person, people involved in caring for them help their families connect with the person and consider whether the symbolism has meaning for that person.

Final gifts

---

1   M. Callanan and P. Kelley, *Final Gifts: Understanding the Special Awareness, Needs, and Communications of the Dying* (Toronto: Bantam Books, 1993).

> A man was dying and called out, "Where's the map?"
>
> The nurse asked the family, "Did your dad work with maps, or were maps important to him?" The family remembered that their dad always liked to know where he was going. The family reassured their dad by telling him that the map was at hand, and he settled without medication.
>
> In another case, a young man who was dying asked his counsellor, "Do you see the old woman sitting in the corner?"
>
> "No, she replied gently, "I don't see her, but tell me what you see."

Although in their book Callanan and Kelley present many case studies in which dying people used symbolic language and saw visions, the authors leave the interpretation of such language and visions up to the families of the dying person. As a PSW, your role is to listen without judgment to their interpretation.

Supporting the family

Witnessing a loved one who is confused, agitated, or paranoid can be extremely upsetting. Caring for someone with delirium can be exhausting for family members. You can help in these ways:

Family need compassion, information, acknowledgment and encouragement

- Acknowledge how stressful it is to witness a loved one experiencing delirium. Assure the family that you have contacted the nurse and the physician.
- Share information on ways to be with a person with delirium, such as walking with them if they want to keep moving.
- Try to orient the person to reality if the person is afraid.
- If the person is comfortable and seems safe in their confusion, demonstrate to the family ways to be with the person in their altered reality.
- Encourage family members who are caring for a dying loved one to try to find ways to care for themselves, for example, by having a nap or going for a walk, while you are in the home.

Carol had suffered a series of small strokes followed by a massive stroke that left her blind, mute, and partially paralyzed. Her large family had gathered around her in the hospital to say their last farewells. Carol's death was marking the passing of a generation in their family: her brother, Charles, had died only the year before, leaving his wife, Victoria. a widow, but consoled by their many grandchildren.

As the physical changes of the last days and hours of death began to occur, Carol's eyes started to track across the room, almost as if she could see something despite her blindness. A smile broke across her face and she lifted her arms and acted as if she were embracing the air above her. Her family stood bewildered, watching this. Carol gestured for a pen and paper, making urgent writing motions as she continued to radiate a joyful smile. When the paper and pen were placed in her hand, she scrawled for a few moments, then relaxed back against the cushions, still smiling as she closed her eyes.

Her family began to weep at she took her last breaths. One of them took up the paper Carol had written on. Barely legible were the words, "Tell Victoria, Charles says hi."

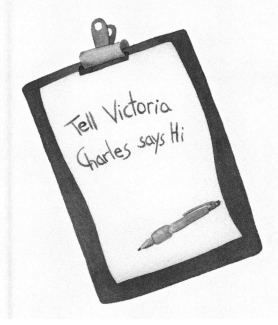

Agitation and/or Restlessness

As death approaches, the dying person may want to be on the move, without knowing what they want to do or where they want to go.

Supporting the dying person

Restlessness may signal that death is near

You, as a PSW, will document restlessness and consider causes, such as pain, a full bladder, constipation, and emotional or spiritual issues. Signs of restlessness should be reported to the nurse promptly. Dealing with restlessness quickly can help ensure that the person will be able to sleep at night. If the person is not confused, guided imagery and other visualization techniques may be helpful.

Supporting the family

It can be exhausting for family when their loved one is unable to settle. These are some things you can do to acknowledge the fatigue and stress the family experiences in dealing with restlessness, as well as the difficulty of caring for someone who is restless and moving all the time:
- Encourage the family to discuss their concerns with the nurse and physician.
- Share information:
  - Explain that restlessness is common in the last days and hours.
  - Provide and model comfort measures to help the person settle, but acknowledge that medications may be needed.

Offer rest breaks to family as they companion the dying person

- Offer family members opportunities to rest and take breaks.

    While I am here would you like to have a nap?

    If we have someone sit with your mom, would you like to get some fresh air or go home and have a shower?

Unresponsiveness

It is normal for people nearing death to respond less to stimulation. Initially they may seem to be sleeping lightly and can be awoken. At other times they may appear to be in a deep sleep and unable to respond to verbal or physical stimuli.

Supporting the dying person

As a PSW, you can reposition the person regularly to protect their skin and increase their comfort. It may be comforting to the person if you continue to talk with them as though they were able to hear you. Introduce yourself when you arrive at their bedside, let them know what you are going to do, and talk as you provide care. Consult with the team to adjust routines as necessary.

Protect skin to increase comfort in an unresponsive person

Supporting the family

The family may have adapted to their loved one not being able to talk and visit but may reach yet another emotional landmark when the person is no longer able to respond at all. You can help by acknowledging the family's sense of loss when their loved one does not respond and is no longer able to talk with them. Family members should be encouraged to continue to talk to the person if they are comfortable doing so. You might say,

> *It is our experience that people can still hear, even when they cannot respond, so feel free to continue to talk as though she were able to hear you. You do not need to speak any louder than normal.*

Encourage family to continue interacting with their loved one – talking, touching and just being there

It is also important to share information. You can help family members explore ways to connect with their loved one by using touch or music, by simply being a quiet presence, or by reminiscing and recalling family stories in the presence of the dying person.

You might suggest the possibility of the dying person talking with other friends or relatives by telephone if they cannot be present. Putting the phone to the person's ear will enable them to have a private, perhaps final conversation, even if the dying person can only listen.

Another way you can be supportive is by teaching the family to position the person, using large and small pillows to support joints and weakened muscles and maintain good body alignment. Massage, touch, and energy work may be relaxing and nurturing to both the giver and the receiver.

Irregular Breathing

When a person is dying, their breathing will usually become irregular, with periods of not breathing (known as apnea). The gaps in breathing can be very long, and family members may find themselves holding their breath and wondering if this is their loved one's last breath. Irregular breathing is not the same as gasping for air. Irregular breathing does not appear to cause discomfort for the dying person.

Supporting the dying person

You can help by positioning the person in a way that supports their breathing and by providing verbal assurance. Some people appear to find comfort in following the voice of a caregiver.

> *That's good, you're doing fine ... just breathe easily.*

When providing care, it may be helpful to model this strategy for the family.

Supporting the family

The family may feel concerned when their loved one's breathing patterns change. It is important to acknowledge that irregular breathing is normal for people in the last days and hours. You might say,

> *Breathing can become very irregular in the last days, with long periods of apnea followed by short or long periods of irregular breathing.*

> *Irregular breathing is normal and in our experience does not appear to be uncomfortable for the dying person.*

You can also provide support by encouraging the family to talk with the nurse if they are concerned that their loved one is uncomfortable. You can share information with the family and nurse in these ways:

- Provide contact information to enable the family to access a support person or the nurse 24 hours a day.
- Explain the difference between what distressed breathing as opposed to irregular breathing might look like. For example, if the person is frowning, looking tense or anxious, or becomes agitated, that may indicate discomfort and the nurse should be contacted.
- Show the family how to freshen and moisten a dry mouth if the person is breathing through their mouth. If the family is interested in helping with care, show them how to use the atomizer and apply lip balm.

Changes in breathing are difficult for family. Ensure they have contact information for a support person

Teaching family to provide mouth care involves them in caring for their loved one

Congested Breathing

I could hear him breathing before I got to the door. He was congested. Moist, rattling sounds occurred with each breath in and with each breath out. He was asleep on his back. He did not respond to my touch and seemed unaware of my presence. I called for the nurse and gave a brief report:

> *I am with Mr. P and his breathing is congested, but he appears comfortable. Can you come and see him now?*

We turned him toward his side. He did not respond. His face was relaxed. I used mouth swabs to remove some of the phlegm from his mouth. When he was on his side, a bit more fluid drained onto the small towel I had put there. In this position, his breathing sounded quieter. We put pillows behind his back, washed his face, and put a fresh towel on his pillow to catch fluid.

Respiratory congestion is common in a person's last days and hours. Moisture from the mouth, throat, or lungs collects in the airways, and the person is unable to clear the secretions by swallowing or coughing. The person can have a little congestion or can become very congested. Most likely, the person will be unresponsive, unaware of, and not distressed by the congestion. Occasionally a dying person will be responsive and uncomfortable or distressed. If medication is given at the first sign of congestion, it often helps decrease secretions.

Respiratory congestion can sound uncomfortable to caregivers

Supporting the dying person

When moist respirations begin, it is best to contact the nurse. You can report the way a person appears in terms of their breathing and position, for example, that the person is relaxed and breathing regularly, agitated, sitting up, lying down, struggling to breathe, gasping for air, attempting to cough, conscious, alert, aware, responsive, or distressed. You can help in these ways:
- Provide a calm and reassuring presence.
- Give frequent mouth care.
- Provide comfort measures for dyspnea.
- Reposition the person to facilitate easier breathing and prevent pooling of secretions in the back of the throat:
  - Elevate or lower the head of the bed.
  - Place pillows under the person's arms to provide support if that makes them more comfortable when they are sitting up.
  - Lay the person flat, turn onto the side on which they are most comfortable, and put a face cloth or small towel under the mouth so that fluids can drain onto the towel. Gently clean the mouth.
  - Help the person into a semi-supine position if they are very congested.
- Record and report the positions in which the person appears to be most comfortable.

Repositioning may help decrease congestion

Supporting the family

The family may be uncomfortable with the sounds of the moist respirations of their loved one. Acknowledging that many people find this type of breathing difficult to hear supports the family. You can also support family members by encouraging them to share their concerns and goals of care with the nurse and physician:

- Encourage the family to contact the nurse if congestion increases or if the person shows signs of discomfort. The nurse can address questions about the use of suctioning to relieve the congestion.
- Share information.
- Make sure the family has easy access to the contact information for the nurse.

Changes in Skin Colour and Temperature

When a person is near death, various changes may occur in the colour and temperature of their skin. Sometimes the skin warms up and cools down again. Cooling of the skin usually begins at the tips of the fingers and toes and gradually works back toward the core of the body. The feet and legs may become bluish, mottled, and cool to the touch. The area where the person's body rests on the mattress may also become bluish.

Skin colour may change and body temperature may cool as death nears

Supporting the dying person

If the person is sweating, you can provide clean clothing and bedding. If the person is cold, you can offer another blanket, but it is important to be aware that the person's skin temperature might change again and should be checked regularly.

Supporting the family

You can help the family in the following ways:
- Acknowledge their concerns about the comfort of their loved one. For example, if the person seems to be cold, it may be helpful to say to the family,

  When a person is dying, they do not appear to feel cold. If we put too many blankets on the bed, the person may begin to sweat.

- Consult with the nurse about the person's physical need to be washed. More frequent washing may be necessary if the person is sweating or is incontinent. Full baths may not be necessary if the person remains clean and dry. The person's preferences about being bathed and touched should be taken into account.
- Share information:
  - Changes in body temperature (e.g., a fever) may indicate an infection or may indicate that the circulatory system is not working well and is shutting down.

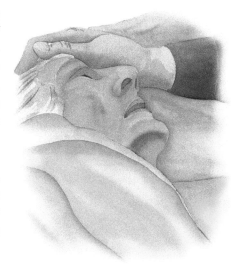

Other Changes As Death Nears

Muscle twitching

Sudden twitching of the muscles in the arms or legs when a person appears to be resting is referred to as "myoclonic" twitching. Metabolic changes may cause this twitching just prior to death. Myoclonic twitching that occurs infrequently or occasionally does not distress the dying person. If such twitching occurs more frequently, it may disturb the person's sleep and may be difficult for the family to witness. When you observe this symptom, you should report it to the nurse for assessment.

Dry eyes

The person's eyes may be open, partially open, or shut during the last days. Seeing a person with only the whites of their eyes showing can be distressing for the family. Remember that families often carry mental images of their loved one's death for a long time after the death. Therefore, it can be helpful to let them know that this is normal. If the distress continues, you can contact the nurse for support.

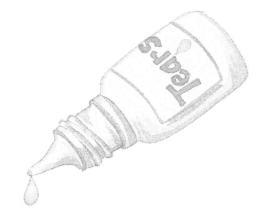

If a person's eyes are open for long periods of time, you can provide comfort by moistening the eyes with artificial tears. Talk with the nurse if the person's eyes appear to be dry. In some cultures, the caregivers place a face cloth over the eyes to keep them closed.

Lack of urinary output and/or bowel and bladder incontinence

Urinary output decreases as kidney function declines in a person's last days. This results in dark, concentrated urine. Urinary incontinence is common among the dying. Some people prefer that a urinary catheter be inserted, while others prefer the use of incontinence pads. It is important to remember that people's preferences may change. You can talk with the person if possible, or speak with the family and the nurse to decide which option is most consistent with the person's preferences.

People sometimes lose control of their bowels as they are dying. It would be practical and may provide a sense of comfort for the person and family to have an incontinence pad in place.

Last Breaths

Last breaths occur in a variety of patterns. Some dying people stop breathing suddenly. Others progress from irregular breathing to deeper breaths that alternate with shallow breaths. Eventually, the person's breathing becomes even shallower, followed by mouth breathing and then none. The person may open their mouth as if to take a last breath.

Sometimes the person's face wrinkles or grimaces at the time of death. This occurs even in people who do not seem to be experiencing any pain. I have been told that adherents of Eastern religions believe that the spirit exits through the head. I wonder if this little grimace is the final little tug of the spirit separating from the body.

When Death Occurs

What You Will See

At the time of death, the person does not have a pulse and does not breathe. Their pupils are enlarged, their eyes are fixed in one position, either open or closed, and their mouth and jaw relax.

The family may look to you to confirm that death has occurred. You may acknowledge that it has:

> *It appears that his heart and his breathing have stopped. I think he has died.*

At this time, you need to follow the care plan and the proper protocol for the care setting and situation. (In some situations, it is appropriate to confirm that you think the person has died. In other settings, you may need to contact the nurse instead.)

People will respond in many different ways when death occurs

When death occurs, you may see the family respond in a variety of ways. You need to remember that each person is unique, and that their responses reflect cultural traditions and family and personal styles and ways of being. It can be difficult to watch people express deep emotion, and you may be tempted to "shush" the person, pat their back, and tell them to breathe or to be quiet. Instead of doing that, you might consider that crying and sobbing may be how the person needs to express their grief. I have never heard of a person who did not eventually stop crying. You may need to breathe deeply yourself so you can relax and be fully present.

Other ways in which people may respond to death are to become silent and withdrawn, get busy with phone calls and organizing the funeral, or reminisce and laugh or cry about old memories. Some people express anger or frustration at the unfairness of the loss, or their perception of a difficult death or a health care system that did not meet their needs.

All of these are normal reactions to death. You do not need to guide, control, or judge people's responses at this time. It is important for you to be present in a calm and supportive way for all involved.

What You Can Do

If there is no signed DNR form in the home or on the chart and the family is not present to refuse cardiopulmonary resuscitation, then you will need to refer to agency or facility policies about responding to death. You may need to call 911.

If death is expected, there is a care plan for the time of death, and there is a signed DNR, then these are the next steps to take:

- Note and record the time of death, when the person's breathing and pulse stopped.
- Breathe. This is not an emergency. Nothing has to happen right away.
- Do not call 911, the ambulance, the police, or the fire department.
- Notify the nurse. The nurse will contact the attending physician. The nurse or physician will pronounce death, unless an "Expected Death Form" has already been completed and a formal pronouncement is not required. If the family is not present, the nurse or physician will notify the family.
- Follow the care plan as prepared.
- Confirm (if this has not already been done) with the family whether any rituals or special preferences regarding care of the body need to be observed. And, if appropriate, create a space in which the rituals can take place.
- Offer the family nourishment, space, and privacy.
- If appropriate, wash or clean the body, position it on the back, place a small pillow under the head, and place the hands either at the person's sides or across the abdomen.
- Tidy the room.
- If the family asks you to remain in the home until the funeral home staff arrive to remove the body, clarify with the nurse how long you may remain with the family.
- If you are alone with the person in a home setting when the death occurs and are not comfortable being alone with the body until the funeral home staff arrive, ask the nurse to join you in the home.

PSWs can record time of death

When death occurs:
- breathe
- record the time
- notify the nurse
- follow the care plan

The family asked us not to put any scented creams or soaps on one of the women we cared for. The family explained that she must go to the next world pure with no smells on her body. We were glad she told us before we used our nice creams on her skin.

Some families bring small bunches of cedar tied with a ribbon and they place it under the pillow of the resident. All the family comes and sits at the bedside until the resident dies. There are usually 4 to 15 people in the room.

> Remember that the goal of HPC is to provide a safe, supportive place in which people can die. The location is not important. It could be a home, an acute care hospital, a long-term care facility, or a hospice unit—a place where the dying person and their caregivers feel safe.

Caring for the Body after Death

Over the past century, the responsibility for washing and preparing the body slowly transitioned from family members to health care and funeral professionals. Interestingly, families are currently re-involving themselves in washing and preparing the body. Regardless of who takes on this responsibility, it is important to consider agency and facility policies for care of the body. These are the steps to follow in caring for the body:

- Position the person lying flat with a pillow under their head.
- Close their eyelids if their eyes are open. If the eyes do not stay closed, you might place a face cloth over the eyelids to hold them closed.
- Wash the face and hands, and the body if the person was incontinent or diaphoretic (sweating).
- Put in the person's dentures if this is important to the family.
- Place an incontinence pad under the buttocks in case of further incontinence.
- Dress the person in a fresh gown or clothing, as appropriate.
- Change soiled linens and arrange the bedding and pillows.
- Follow procedures set out for and the family's wishes with respect to the removal of personal effects, such as jewellery.
- Prepare the body as respectfully as you would if the family were present.

Follow and respect family wishes when caring for the body

About three or four hours after a person dies, chemical changes cause stiffening of the body, known as rigor mortis. For this reason, caring for the body in the first few hours after death is easier than waiting until the body cools and become less flexible. The work of digestion continues after death, which means that gases may escape the body when it is being washed or moved. These sounds are normal.

When Maude died her family respectfully fulfilled her last wishes down to the last detail. I assisted with bathing her and then brought tea to the family as they dressed her and shared stories of her life. They honoured her glamour and style as they dressed her in her traditional Scottish regalia (which she had specifically chosen for this occasion). Then the granddaughter applied bright red nail polish and the daughter applied Maude's makeup.

Creating a Special Space

As a person is dying and following their death, there may be opportunities to create a special or sacred space, and a moment in time dedicated to the person who has died and to their life. The family may want the opportunity to observe or create rituals or traditions, or to be in the moment in a way that brings meaning and understanding.

Follow the family's lead regarding rituals at time of death

On rituals

Rituals can help create a sacred or special place. They can honour and show respect for the person who has died, and respect for traditions, beliefs, and heritage. Angeles Arrien, a cultural anthropologist, author, and teacher, suggests that rituals can support and strengthen, balance and comfort:

> *Ritual provides the bridge between inner and outer worlds, and creates a context of connecting to our souls. The result of all ritual is increased balance, strength, energy, and comfort.*[2]

Rituals can help people find meaning, grasp the significance of what has occurred, and transition to a new place in grief. Rituals can create memories.

Although people often think of rituals as ceremonies and services that are repeated events, or events that are offered routinely, rituals can also be behaviours that are done only one time for this person but—when considered as part of the human family over the millennia—are repeated. Rituals can also be considered to be those activities that are used to create a special moment.

Religious or spiritual rituals include praying, chanting, smudging, communion, blessings, lighting candles, ringing bells, singing, opening windows, covering mirrors, touching or not touching the body, reminiscing, and sharing stories. Rituals that involve caring for the body may include bathing the person, rubbing the skin with special oils, dressing the body in particular clothing, washing the feet, and placing flowers in the hair or a memento in the hands or on the chest. Rituals can be as simple as thoughtfully covering the person's face when the body is placed in the casket. Rituals can last for moments or extend over days. Rituals may be performed by spiritual leaders or offered by family members. Rituals may be passed down through the centuries or created in the moment.

---

2 Angeles Arrien, quoted in Louis LaGrand, *Gifts from the Unknown: Using Extraordinary Experiences to Cope with Loss and Change* (San Jose: Author's Choice Press, 2001), 156.

If the family has not yet explored the idea of rituals or traditions, you might want to ask a few questions and open the door to exploring the idea. Be mindful to ask in a neutral manner that allows the family to decline. You might ask,

Are there any important traditions in your family, culture, or religious community that you would like to honour or observe?

Explore rituals at time of death by asking family these questions

Are there any restrictions on touching the body or who is supposed to bathe the body?

Is there anything that I can do that would help you carry out a ritual that is important to you at this time?

If the family identifies traditions or rituals that are important to them, it may be helpful to:
- Create a comfortable, private area
- Remove medical equipment, linens, and health care supplies
- Tidy the room and empty the garbage
- Put fresh linen on the bed and/or tidy the bed

If death occurs in acute or long-term care settings (as in the following story), you can still explore with the family their preferences for use of ritual and then work with the nurses and management to create a special space in which the family can be with the deceased.

The gentleman came into the emergency department critically ill. The doctors told the family he had only an hour or two to live. The man and his family were devout Buddhists. They requested space to perform a traditional seven-hour chant.

The manager did not want the department disrupted, but she wanted to respect the family's wishes. A private area was needed. She remembered the large storeroom at the end of the hallway, away from the main part of the unit. The room was hastily emptied, cleaned, and tidied. The dying man was moved in. He died peacefully with all his family around him. The chanting began. No one was disturbed.

The nurses were so moved by this event they requested that this room be set aside for people who are dying and their families. The room has been a great resource for families, and it also provides a place for the staff to pay their respects to the dying person and their family. For the nurses who work in emergency and who all too often witness traumatic deaths, this room has been a source of comfort for them as well.

Rituals can develop spontaneously. As a PSW, you can step back and watch as the family finds ways to create ritual that has meaning to them and brings them together.

When Yetta was dying, my brothers found a piece of driftwood and a rope on the beach that inspired them to build a coffin. My brothers and husband designed and built a beautiful but simple pine coffin. In fact, the coffin was so beautiful that it was not used in the cremation; instead it will be recycled for future loved ones who want to share in this treasure. The idea of reusing, recycling, and being environmentally friendly added to the strength of the rituals of caring for Yetta's body after death.

While my brothers were building the coffin, my sister (a fabric artist like Yetta) and I designed and sewed a shroud to provide a beautiful wrap for Yetta's body. The materials came from Yetta's studio and included silk fabrics that my sister had silk-screened, and, like the coffin, the shroud was a beautiful work of art. The coffin and shroud both reflected the creativity that Yetta had passed on to us. These were personal works of art but still met the legal requirements of the province.

As we engaged in building the coffin and sewing the shroud, we were also involved in one of life's oldest rituals, that of caregiving. We came together to build, to sew, and to give care. We left with powerful memories and images that remain with us.

The following story describes a death that was difficult and a PSW who used rituals to create a space for the family to come together in a healing way.

The death had been difficult. In the end, the man tried to climb out of bed and died in the process. The family was exhausted, sobbing, and distressed. The PSW phoned the nurse to notify her of the death, and asked for help immediately to support the family and prepare the body.

At the family's request the PSW provided tea and helped them settle in the living room. The nurse arrived and together the nurse and the PSW went to care for the man who had died. They entered the room, shut the door, took some deep breaths, and opened the window to let fresh air fill the room. They played his music quietly.

The nurse began by asking the PSW what she knew about the man who had died. The PSW began to tell the story of a wonderful man, his fascinating life, and how he was much loved by his devoted family. Together the nurse and the PSW talked back and forth while they gently washed the body, changed the sheets, cleaned and tidied the room, and threw out the garbage. Then they stood at the bedside, hand in hand, in a moment of silence.

The PSW and the family picked a few of the man's much-loved flowers from his garden and gathered together around the bedside. In this space the family reminisced and shared memories and stories.

The ritual of caregiving brought order out of chaos and prepared a space for the family to come together to honour their loved one.

On making meaning

Sometimes, by being attentive to nature, people discover ways to give meaning to events that occur at the time of death or during the dying process. By listening to and watching the natural world, they find meaning in an event that others may not have noticed. And in making the meaning, they create a sacred, special, or healing space, and open the door to larger possibilities. In some ways, the act of listening and attending could be considered a ritual, or it could be considered an alternative to ritual.

Be open to opportunities to make meaning during the dying process

Examples people have shared about finding meaning in nature at the time of a death are a ray of sunshine falling across the bed of the dying person, a bird singing loud and clear nearby, a gust of wind blowing through the window, and eagles soaring overhead as a First Nation elder died.

A woman was dying at home. The deer that normally passed by the window each morning stopped by the sliding glass doors and looks into her room. The deer became a frequent visitor. On the last day the deer brought her two fawns with her. They knelt by the window, not moving, waiting. When the woman died, the deer left. The family was moved by their presence, and comforted by what they felt was a unique and special experience.

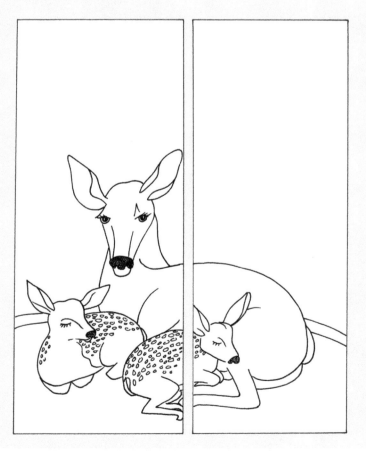

The following story is shared by Lindsay Borrows, who writes of the rituals in her Anishinaabe community.

When someone is dying, many of the older people know how to listen to the dying person's breath and they can tell when the person only has a few days left on the earth. There are signs in nature as well, which indicate when someone is close to dying. When my great-grandpa passed away, his friend saw four ducks circling in a pond. Then he looked up and, as if in reflection of the ducks, four birds circled overhead. He felt this was not a coincidence but was a message with important symbolism of the circle, the number four, and the birds. The circle represents the continuity of life, that endings bring new beginnings. The number four speaks to each of the four directions, and when someone passes they head home to the north—giiwedin. Birds are the messengers of death. He immediately went home and his wife informed him that my great-grandpa had died. He was not surprised, knowing that nature can provide comfort and closure.

It is possible to create a space that allows the family to observe or create rituals or to be in a moment in a way that brings meaning or understanding to the death. As a PSW you can facilitate this process.

Supporting

Supporting the family

The family of a person who has died may feel exhausted, hungry, thirsty, tired, emotional, and/or tearful. They may not remember what they are supposed to do following the death and may need to be reminded. As the PSW, you can help in these ways:

- Offer nourishment, such as a hot drink and a snack. Companioning someone through to death can be tiring. Physical nourishment provides the family with a break before taking care of the body. It can also provide space for spiritual support.

  PSWs can provide physical and emotional nourishment to family

- Invite individual people or the family to sit with their loved one. You might say things like the following:

  Some people like to have some quiet time with their loved one following death. Would you like to have some time together as a group or some time alone with your dad?

  Some people don't really know what they want to do or say when they sit with their loved one after the person has died. Some people talk as though the person is still alive and able to hear them. Others prefer to sit quietly in prayer or meditation.

  I can sit with you if that would help you feel more comfortable.

It is also important to consider the needs of people who are not present at the time of death and those coming from out of town. You might say to the family,

Sometimes people who were not present at the time of death want an opportunity to see or have time with the loved one's body. You can keep the body at home for a few more hours, or you can arrange for a visitation at the funeral home. What would you like to do?

In the minutes and hours following death, the physical presence of the deceased can help to make the death "real." For those who may have watched their loved one struggle in the last days and hours, it may be a time to see the body "at peace." Sitting with the deceased person can help people understand in a new way, perhaps a deeper way, that the death really has occurred. Caring for the body, as described previously, can help to create ritual and meaning in the experience.

Some facilities require that the room be ready as soon as possible for the next person to be admitted. This happens in acute care, emergency care, and long-term care facilities. If the family members feel very strongly about being with the deceased, you may need to advocate on their behalf. If hospital policy is not flexible enough to accommodate the needs of the family, the family may want to arrange time for visitation at the funeral home.

Family may need the health care team to advocate for more time with the deceased

It can be difficult to find an appropriate space for rituals in some facilities. Fortunately, the cultural competency of health care personnel has improved over the past decades. Sometimes some creativity can help the health care team come up with options that work for the family and allow them to observe the rituals important to them.

In the Creative Arts studio, we give the family something that has been worked on by their loved one (ie. a bag or an apron) to have as a keepsake in memory of them.
—Sylvia Mills

A young man was dying. His parents, who were of the Baha'i faith, arrived from the Middle East just days before his death. In addition to their grief, they were in a foreign country with no support. Staff explored with the family what practices would be common in their home community at such a time. With permission from the family, the staff contacted the local Baha'i community and invited them to the unit. The community prayed with the family around the bed and created a special feast. At the time of death, the mother took off her beautiful shawl and placed it over her son's face. When the body was removed from the unit, the shawl remained in place, and the body bag, in keeping with the family's wishes, was not closed. This family felt supported.

Supporting other residents

In long-term care homes and hospices, the residents often come to know each other. These people also need support when a person who lived among them dies. In long-term care facilities, the residents closest to the deceased are sometimes invited into the room to say their farewells before the body is removed. In one hospice residence, the staff, residents, and family developed a ritual that works well for them. It is described below.

Other residents may want an opportunity to say good bye

When someone dies, a staff member notifies each resident (and family who are present) of the death. Each resident can come to the bedside of the deceased to say goodbye. We do not share details about the person who died, but we listen to the residents and let them tell us how they are feeling. We assure them that … their feelings are valued.

A small lamp on a shelf in the hallway is lit. A member of the staff places a card with the person's name on it next to the lamp. Families may put flowers or a photograph alongside.

Once a week tea is served and residents are invited to remember the person who died. Often families attend this tea. Staff members try to attend. There are stories, maybe a song, sometimes a prayer, tears, hugs, and smiles, and usually there is some laughter. One time the person who died left a letter to be read to everyone—he said he did not want to miss his special memorial.

Supporting the staff

Just as the residents need time to say goodbye and honour and remember the person who has died, the staff may also appreciate the opportunity to say goodbye. Rituals can help the staff acknowledge their own grief about the death of yet another resident, may help them develop a sense of satisfaction in having provided good care, and may support them as they continue to provide compassionate care to the dying.

Debriefing with Staff

In the story below, PSW Jackie McDonald, a participant and leader in the Quality Palliative Care in Long Term Care research project, shares what the staff at the care home where she works do after the death of a resident.[3]

Immediately after a person dies, we open a window. We believe this freshens the room; some believe it is a pathway out for the spirit. A staff member puts a butterfly on the frame of the door to let everyone know that the resident has died. We tidy up the resident if needed, tidy the bed, put all bed rails down, and give the family privacy to say their goodbyes.

Staff come to say goodbye to the family, because we are losing them when we lose the resident.

When the family leaves, we say goodbye to our resident.

When the funeral home staff come, we place a dignity quilt over the body bag, and a member of our staff walks the resident's body out to the funeral van and returns with the quilt.

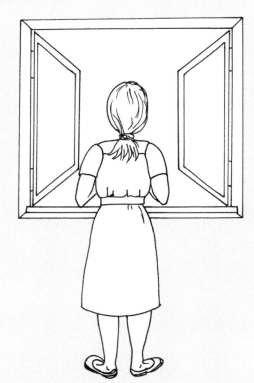

We place a decorated memory box on the bed of the resident. On the lid of the box is a beautiful poem and information on grief counselling from one of our community partners, which also donates the boxes to our home.

We put a sympathy card on our table in the staff room for staff to sign and write stories about our resident. Within a week, it is mailed to the family. It is a beautiful moment when you look down at this card and see the many stories and signatures of the many people who have worked hard to make sure this resident left this world with dignity and love.

— Jackie McDonald

3 Palliative Alliance (Quality Palliative Care in Long Term Care) Communication, http://www.palliativealliance.ca/communication.

Jackie McDonald shared with me her experience of leading staff debriefing sessions after the death of a resident.[4]

A few years ago, almost half of our residents died in one year. We called it the "pancake effect," with one death on top of another. There was no way to grieve or say goodbye. Staff could not always go to the funeral, as they were working. We decided to have a peer-to-peer debriefing to care for ourselves after a person died. Management has supported this initiative from the start. As a PSW, I was trained to lead these debriefings.

We try to have a debriefing within hours of a death. Staff gather for 15 to 20 minutes. Attendance is always voluntary—people attend because they want or need to. Sometimes there are a few people while at other times there is a full room with someone from all departments. There is no hierarchy, just co-workers remembering our special resident. The debriefing is led by a personal support worker, which helps people feel equal in the debriefing. There is no expectation that you have to talk.

We use the acronym INNPUT to give structure to the meeting.

*I—**Information** about resident: name, how long in home, and any other pertinent details.*

*N—**Need to do.** What can we do to help staff finish the shift, get through the day or the week. Staff members may need a hug, reassurance, or recognition that the person was very special to them.*

*N—**Need to say.** Exchange stories about what made this person special to you. What was important to you about the resident and/or their family?*

*P—**Plan for self-care.** What will you do to help yourself? Go for a long walk, go to the funeral, sign the card for the family?*

*U—**Understanding.** We need to understand everyone grieves in a different way. Understand that it is all right to feel sad, to be angry, and/or to feel as if something is missing. These are all parts of the grieving process. We need to understand that these feelings will pass. To understand that it's all right to seek help through each other, access the Employee Assistance Program, or your own counsellor/spiritual person.*

*T—**Thank you.** We acknowledge and thank everyone for their contributions to the well-being of our resident, family, each other, and themselves.*
— Jackie McDonald

---

4 Palliative Alliance (Quality Palliative Care in Long Term Care), *Peer Led Debriefing Toolkit: Guidelines for Promoting Effective Grief Support Among Front Line Staff*, http://www.palliativealliance.ca/assets/files/Alliance_Reources/Org_Change/Toolkit_Sept4th_BUNNY-_Jan_7-_Final.pdf.

In a care facility, the information about a death and a debriefing can occur relatively easily. In community care situations, a debriefing can be more complicated to set up. As a PSW, you can:

Death affects everyone. Take care of yourself by debriefing after the person dies

- Ask the office to inform you when someone you worked closely with has died
- Identify when you need to debrief after a death
- Request help when you need support
- Develop a buddy system that provides you with an opportunity to debrief with a colleague while maintaining confidentiality
- Develop a personal ritual to remember and honour the person who has died, to say goodbye, and to let the person go

When a client dies, I open a window, say goodbye, and stand in silence for a moment.

Preparing to Transfer the Body

Each agency or facility has policies on how to care for the body and preparing it for transport. PSWs need to be familiar with these policies and follow them.

This is what occurs in most hospitals and long-term care facilities:

Family may feel the finality of death again when the body leaves. Prepare them for this experience.

- The PSW or nurse dresses the body in a gown and covers it with a sheet, leaving the face exposed.
- In hospitals, some means of identification (e.g., an armband), including the person's name and birth date, is secured around the person's wrist.
- The funeral home staff put the body in a body bag, close the zipper, place the body on a stretcher, and transport the body to the funeral home.
- The nurse often calls the funeral home when the body is ready to be removed, but the family can complete this task if they want to.
- The family may want to accompany the body to the funeral van.
- In a home setting, the family may request that the zipper be left partially open and that the face be exposed. This provides an opportunity for the family to kiss the person, put a flower on the chest, or observe some other ritual in saying goodbye.

It may be helpful to inform the family that the removal of the body can often feel as final as the death itself. The family may want to be present when the body is removed, or may prefer to go to another room or leave before the body is taken away.

I work in a facility where 90% of the residents have advanced dementia. The recreation therapist worked with a large group of the residents to make a simple but beautiful quilt. This quilt is laid over each body as it is transferred to the funeral van. It is our way to collectively honour the resident.

When Death Is Sudden and Unexpected

It is hoped that preparing for death will remove a sense of crisis when death does occur. If people have not prepared for the death or the death is sudden and unexpected, then there is a need to respond quickly. If you discover a person has died suddenly and unexpectedly, follow agency policy.

When a sudden and unexpected death occurs in a home,
- Call 911
- Notify the nurse and follow instructions
- Leave the person and the room as you found it
- Remain with the body until the paramedics arrive

When death occurs in a long-term or acute care setting,
- Inform the nurse
- Leave the patient and room as you found it
- Record what you observed

The Role of the Coroner When Death Is Sudden

When a person's death is sudden, unexpected, or occurs within 24 hours of admission to a hospital, the coroner is notified. The role of the coroner is to confirm the identity of the person who died and the probable cause and time of death. The coroner classifies the death as natural, accidental, suicide, homicide, or undetermined.

The coroner is called when death is sudden and unexpected

If the coroner determines that the death is due to natural causes, usually no further investigation takes place. If there are concerns about the identity of the person or the cause of death, then the coroner will investigate. If you are the person who discovered the dead person and the coroner is involved, you may be interviewed and asked to describe what you saw. The coroner's role is to protect the public and help identify factors that contribute to preventable causes of death. The coroner also helps family and survivors by providing links to resources and support.

The Home Funeral Movement

An increasing number of families are choosing to provide care for their deceased loved ones. This may include any combination of the following: making the coffin, sewing a shroud to wrap the body in, washing and dressing the body, keeping the body in the home for a longer than usual period after death, registering the death, transporting the body to the church, crematorium, or burial ground, and helping to bury the body.

This growing interest in "do-it-yourself" death care relates not only to caring for the deceased, but also usually addresses caring for the person and family before death. This emerging field is giving rise to new types of caregivers: death doulas and death midwives. Like the HPC teams, the doulas and midwives provide holistic, family- and person-oriented care for the dying and deceased. Funeral celebrants lead services and rituals that are personalized to the beliefs and style of the deceased and their families.

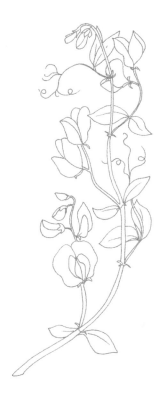

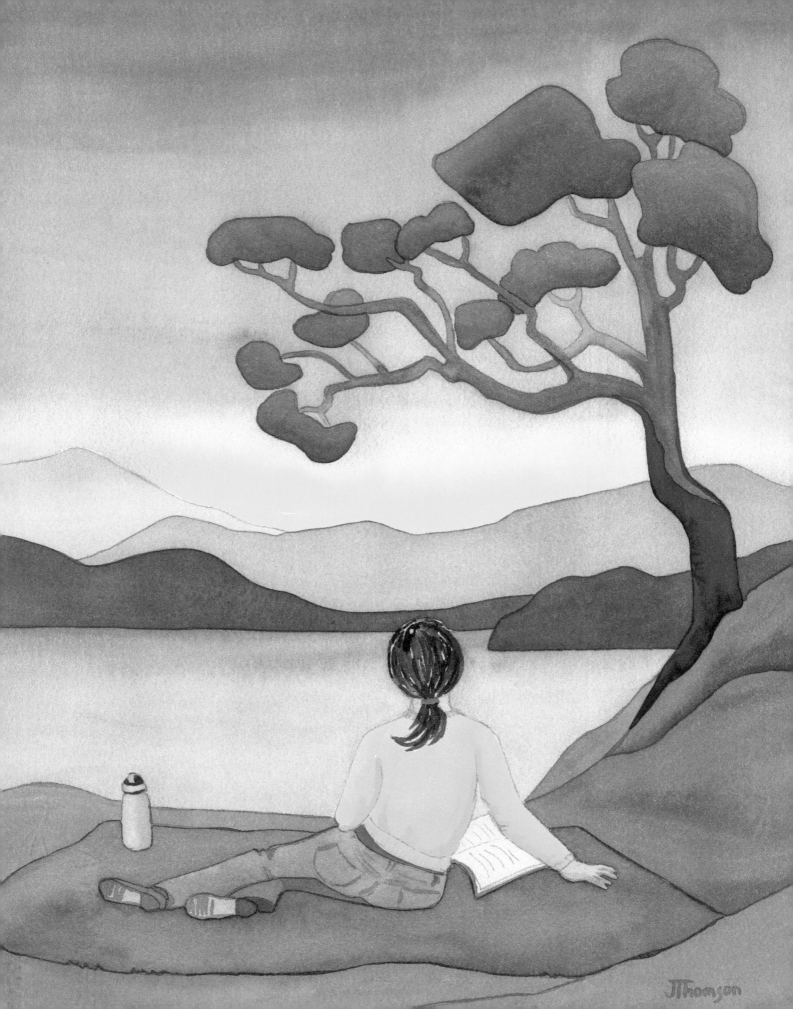

7

Caring for *You!*

Providing Care for the Dying Will Change You

Caring for the dying will touch you and change you. In her book *Kitchen Table Wisdom: Stories That Heal,* Rachel Naomi Remen says,

> The expectation that we can be immersed in suffering and loss daily and not be touched by it is as unrealistic as expecting to be able to walk through water without getting wet.[1]

There are consequences, both positive and negative, to providing palliative care. Being with people during their dying process may enhance your enjoyment of living, increase your appreciation of simple things, strengthen your ability to empathize, and increase your awareness of the challenges that people experience. These benefits may increase your capacity to care and may inspire you to face your own challenges with renewed strength and determination.

Care for yourself so that you can provide care for the dying

On the negative side, there may be times when your work and the sorrow you witness leave you grieving, sad, and feeling exhausted. You may find yourself grieving the dying person's losses as though they were your own. You may feel guilty that you are mobile while the person you care for is immobile, that you are living while they are dying.

The purpose of this chapter is to stress the importance of caring for *you*! You do invaluable work, but you need to care for yourself as well as you care for others. You need to develop strong social support networks, and learn and grow through education, supervision, counselling, and coaching. Simple self-care strategies will help you refuel. When you are fatigued (and you will be), step back, reflect, shake things up a bit, and get some extra support.

---

1   N.R. Remen, *Kitchen Table Wisdom: Stories That Heal* (New York: Putnam, 1997), 52.

Self-Care—Buffering the Effects of Caregiving

Caregivers must take time for self-care to prevent burnout or "compassion fatigue." Françoise Mathieu, a mental health counsellor and compassion fatigue specialist, is the author of *The Compassion Fatigue Workbook: Creative Tools for Transforming Compassion Fatigue and Vicarious Traumatization*,[2] which is aimed at helping health care providers care for themselves. She also works with organizations to help them develop ways to better support their staff. I am honoured by the author's significant contribution to this chapter and thank her for it.

How does compassion fatigue develop?

The term "compassion fatigue" describes the emotional and physical exhaustion that can occur when the caregiver is unable to refuel and regenerate quickly enough to meet the emotional and physical demands of the work. The type of work, the repetition of doing the work day after day and year after year, and witnessing suffering contribute to compassion fatigue. In addition to the demands of the work itself, challenges such as workload issues, staffing problems, and policies and procedures can cause compassion fatigue.

These behaviours are signs that a person may be developing compassion fatigue

Self-care can help you withstand the negative effects of caring for the dying and benefit from the positive effects. Without the buffer provided by self-care, caregivers may lose their capacity to provide excellent care for the dying. For example, caregivers with compassion fatigue may be impatient, cynical, and/or irritable, be less sensitive to or less able to empathize with people, be neglectful or dismissive of suffering, and be rough with clients and colleagues.

---

2 F. Mathieu, *The Compassion Fatigue Workbook: Creative Tools for Transforming Compassion Fatigue and Vicarious Traumatization* (New York: Taylor & Francis Group, 2012).

Checking In: Signs of Compassion Fatigue

People who care for the dying differ greatly in the type and amount of self-care they need. Your needs for self-care may also change as you develop skills and learn from caregiving experiences.

Françoise Mathieu developed a chart of thoughts and feelings that caregivers can use to assess their self-care needs in relation to compassion fatigue. On the basis of their thoughts and feelings and behaviours, caregivers can assess which zone on the chart they are in. Mathieu uses the colours of a traffic light to indicate when caregivers are safe to go ahead (green), when they may proceed cautiously (yellow), and when to stop (red). Although the colours indicate zones, it is useful to think of the zones as a continuum from health to severe immobilizing fatigue. The goal is to encourage caregivers to use strategies that help them remain healthy and in the green zone.

Your self-care needs may increase when you provide care for the dying

You can use the chart on the following two pages to assess where you are on the continuum from health and enthusiasm to severe compassion fatigue.

Checking In: Signs of Compassion Fatigue

Green Zone	Yellow Zone
Feeling	**Feeling**
You are at your absolute best: well rested, organized, and feeling on top of the world.	You are not coping as well. Things are not as smooth as they were.
You are enthusiastic about your work and excited to go to work each day. You love it.	Perhaps you are more tired, more irritable. You are starting to feel overworked, and perhaps overwhelmed by the demands placed on you.
	You once loved the work you did, but now you are bored when people tell you their problems. You ignore problems that you cannot fix and ask only those questions that will result in a discussion that is easy and positive.
Thinking	**Thinking**
Life is good. Work is good. Let's go!	*I loved my work, for years I loved it. Then with all the cut backs, fewer staff, fewer resources, no flexibility to switch shifts or take time off, no vacation relief ... the recent policy changes, I am starting to hate work. And not only am I mad with management, I don't even feel the same joy in caring for the people I am assigned to care for. I hate it. And I hate myself for not working with the joy that I always worked with.*
Reflection	**Reflection**
Are you in the Green Zone?	Have you been in the Yellow Zone? What does the Yellow Zone feel like for you?
If you are not in the Green Zone now, can you remember being there?	Sometimes people live in this place feeling overloaded and are barely aware of it.
What does being in the Green Zone feel like for you? Take a minute to feel it and enjoy the feeling of energy and inspiration.	What brought you to this place of increasing fatigue?
	Do you have any physical symptoms of fatigue? chronic pain? headaches? back pain?
	What about emotional symptoms? irritability? tearfulness?
In your life, how do you care for yourself so that you can stay in the Green Zone?	Some people find it more difficult to take care of themselves in the Yellow Zone: they eat more junk food, exercise less, and get less sleep. What are your health behaviours when you are in the Yellow Zone?
	Can you imagine anything that might push you further toward the Red Zone?
	What can you do to move back to the Green Zone?

Red Zone

Feeling

You feel unable to cope. If you can even fall asleep, you wake up wondering how you can get out of bed, care for the kids, go to work, and care for those people you are assigned to for one more day.

You are not interested in hearing about any problems, advocating for anyone who needs any changes, and hope that no one asks anything extra of you.

Your co-workers, if they are not aware, should be aware to leave you alone and not ask for your help.

Or:

You are frequently tearful at the drop of a hat. You feel angry if someone even looks at you.

Someone suggested you take a stress leave, but you can't imagine how much work it might take to make that happen.

You wonder if it would be easier to quit your job.

You have never been depressed before, but wonder if this is what depression looks and feels like.

Thinking

I didn't realize I had a problem. I knew I was tired. I knew I was frustrated ... But one day I woke up and I could not get out of bed. I could not care for my kids, or go to work. I was totally and completely immobilized. My partner took me to the doctor. She signed me off work for a month. I could not believe it. A month ... surely, I would feel better in a few days. Nevertheless, a month went, and the numbness was just wearing off and the pain was just beginning. It took me nine months before I was back at work.

Reflection

Have you been in the Red Zone? Are you in the Red Zone now?

What does the Red Zone feel like for you?

If you are in the Red Zone now, speak to your doctor or counsellor.

Get support from the Employee Assistance Program.

Is there anything that you can do today to nourish yourself?

Can you connect with a friend or a supervisor to talk about how you are doing?

Can you ask friends/family for support to help you get professional support and develop some strategies to get out of the Red Zone?

Self-Care Strategies for Caregivers

The following strategies may help prevent compassion fatigue and help you refuel, refocus, care for yourself, and keep you in the Green Zone. If you are emotionally exhausted, you may need to seek professional help, as well as integrate self-care strategies into your daily routine.

Developing Self-Awareness

Personal reflection, as discussed in Chapter 1, can be a valuable strategy for exploring personal issues and understanding your needs. Writing in a journal or talking with a friend or counsellor are other useful reflective strategies.

Considering the following may help develop your reflective skills:

Self-care means checking on your energy levels and emotions

1. Mentally scan your body and "listen" to what it tells you about how you feel.
   - How is your energy level?
   - How does your body communicate to you when you are feeling tense, stressed, hurt, angry, resentful, or other emotions? For example, do you get rashes, an upset stomach, pain, headaches, or other physical discomfort?
2. Reflect on how you process your emotions.
   - What do you do when you feel anger? Do you talk about it, exercise, explode, or swallow your anger?
   - What do you do when you are sad?
   - What you do when you feel overwhelmed?
3. Listen to your conversations.
   - What do you talk about?
   - How do you describe your work, your colleagues, the people you care for?
4. When you start to feel stressed, examine your decision making. Do you
   - Agree to do things you don't have time for?
   - Take on more responsibilities?
   - Drink alcohol or eat excessively?
   - Cancel self-care appointments, doctor's appointments, haircuts, and other appointments relating to you?

Remembering Your Boundaries

For PSWs, establishing and maintaining boundaries when providing care for the dying can be difficult for many reasons. The dying person or their family may ask you to do tasks or answer questions that are outside of your scope of practice. The person and family may begin to think of you as part of the extended family rather than as a caregiver who has been hired to provide care. Your employer's expectations about your work may be different from the family's.

Maintaining therapeutic boundaries is part of effective self-care

Your stress level will increase if you do not have clear boundaries. Setting boundaries may become even more difficult when you are stressed and fatigued.

Blurred boundaries lead to emotional exhaustion and can be a sign of work over-load. If you are near the Red Zone, boundaries become more and more muddled. Some people become very rigid when their energy is depleted; others may become excessively flexible and work outside the limits of their job description because they feel sorry for the person they are caring for.

Strategies for maintaining boundaries

Strategies like those below may help you maintain boundaries:

- Listen to what you say about your work at work and at home.

    I am not hired to bring the family tea, and I don't do it. I am not staying after work one more day. They cannot expect us to stay!

- Talk with a trusted colleague, mentor, or supervisor when you want to provide care outside of work hours.

    The client's wife needs help just as much as he does. I have reported this to the team, but so far the wife has not received any help. I have time between appointments, so I help her get washed and dressed. Last week on my day off, I did errands for them. I would like to talk to you about this and about setting boundaries.

- Review your job description and employee policies to remind yourself what is expected of you.
- Write about boundaries in your journal.

Boundaries are especially difficult to maintain when you live and work in a very small community. Coaching or counselling are increasingly available via phone and may help you get some perspective on local issues without breaking confidentiality.

Explore strategies to help you maintain boundaries

Boundaries are especially difficult when working in a small community.

Developing a Strong Social Support Network

Having social support at home and at work can help prevent compassion fatigue.

Strategies for developing a strong support network

These are some things you can do to build your network:

- Develop relationships with people away from work, as well as with colleagues and supervisors at work.
- Seek out like-minded colleagues for conversation and inspiration.
- Develop a buddy system (with two or three people) or study group and meet to explore relevant topics. Together you could
    - Explore self-care
    - Debrief and learn from stories of caregiving (while honouring confidentiality)
    - Study a chapter of *The Compassion Fatigue Workbook*[3]

    If you cannot connect with other people in person, consider meeting on the phone or joining an online support group.
- Talk with a partner, friend, or roommate about the work you do, the fatigue you experience, and what is helpful when you are feeling very depleted.
- Have fun! Make time for fun with friends!

Develop a strong social network

Strategies for support when working alone in the community

It is more difficult to meet and interact with other caregivers when you work in home and community care settings. In these situations, it is even more important to create a support network for yourself. These strategies may be helpful:

- Find a few colleagues with whom you can connect regularly for a snack, phone call, power walk, or to share some common interest.
- Meet with your employer to discuss these topics:
    - Your desire to do an excellent job, continue to learn and grow, maintain your health, and prevent compassion fatigue
    - Your desire to connect with colleagues
    - Guidelines on confidentiality
    - Ways that your agency supports debriefing, ongoing education, peer support, and workload management
    - Your offer to help organize a room in your workplace where the PSWs can gather to talk, eat, and have education sessions. You might suggest to your employer that strong social networks help prevent compassion fatigue, and that having a room for this purpose would be a good investment

When you work alone in the community, develop ways to meet with colleagues

Strategies for support when working in a negative or toxic workplace

You may notice that compassion fatigue often leads to a negative or toxic workplace. Instead of working together and supporting one another, staff may turn against each other, gossip, backbite, bully others, and develop an "us versus them"

---

3   F. Mathieu, *The Compassion Fatigue Workbook*.

attitude. Here are some things you can do to try to prevent this happening in your work environment:

- Commit to avoid starting or spreading gossip.
- Develop relationships with colleagues who are positive and are interested in being constructive and proactive at work.
- Express gratitude openly and anonymously (e.g., write a note, put a flower on someone's desk).

Self-care strategies for working in an uncomfortable or toxic work environment

Learning

Education is one of my very favourite self-care strategies. I am inspired by new ideas and use the creative process to apply what I learned to my practice. I am also thrilled when I learn skills that enable me to do my job better. Being prepared to do your work and having the necessary education can help prevent compassion fatigue. Expand your knowledge to keep up with the expanding scope of practice, new developments, and changes in policy and practice. No basic program can prepare you to do everything that you will do as a PSW.

Strategies for learning

These are some strategies to help you increase your knowledge:

- Reflect on what type of education and learning makes you excited.
- Try to identify what topics you need to learn more about.
- Watch for and take advantage of educational opportunities, such as workshops, conferences, and lunchtime lectures in your area.
- Request feedback from supervisors or a trusted mentor.
- Meet with colleagues and supervisors to develop educational opportunities.
- Search for educational opportunities online (you can do this at home, in your pyjamas, with the cat on your lap!).
- Offer to help with research projects and champion skill development in areas that you are passionate about. Believe in your ability to influence care.

Learning new skills and activities can be very effective forms of self-care

Refuelling

Refuel yourself using the many self-care strategies that nourish you and your spirit. Choose strategies that are meaningful to you and will energize you. You need to schedule them into your life regularly enough to keep yourself fuelled up. The important part of refuelling is to make the effort even though sometimes you do not feel you have the time or energy to do so. It is then that these strategies are most important to your well-being. Sometimes the most helpful thing you can do is call on your social support network to work together on refuelling.

Some ways to refuel are listed below. The list is not comprehensive and does not provide instruction. If an idea interests you, then explore it further using books, websites, and courses to guide you.

Eat food that nourishes you

Keeping your body in good working condition assists with developing emotional resilience

PSWs are often very busy during the day, so it is easy to fall into the pattern of grabbing a quick bite on the fly. Try to prepare healthy, easy-to-eat, nutritious snacks in advance, take them to work, and enjoy them throughout the day. Avoid turning to sugar and carbohydrates for a quick fix. (I say this as I dream of my favourite dark chocolate ice-cream!)

Drink water

Drinking water is a bit like having a shower: it cleanses your insides just as a shower cleanses your outside. Water increases energy, relieves fatigue, helps cleanse your body of waste, and boosts the immune system. Keep a water bottle with you at work, and try to develop a habit of drinking water between clients and at breaks.

Exercise regularly and stretch often

Exercise for at least 30 minutes a day! (The first 30 minutes of exercise provides the most benefit.) If you work in isolation, you may find it helpful to exercise with another person. If you work in a group, you may prefer to exercise on your own. If the physical care you provide requires a lot of strength and exertion, consider attending a fitness class to strengthen the muscles you use regularly at work, or get a group together and consult with a personal trainer to develop an exercise routine that will increase your strength and so help prevent injuries.

Stretching is another good practice. It can increase your flexibility, range of motion, circulation, and energy level, as well as reduce stress, muscle tension, and lower back pain.

I do yoga as a way to relax. At work, when I feel my muscles tighten I find a quiet space. I breathe deeply and stretch the area that is tight. Doing this I am able to prevent my back muscles from going into spasm.

Sleep well

Sleep well and sleep long enough. Integrate "sleep hygiene" habits in the hour or so before you go to bed: go for a walk, have a warm bath, pray or meditate, read a soothing book, listen to calming music, and avoid using devices with backlit screens (e.g., tablets and smartphones) at least for the hour before you go to bed. If you work night shifts or have difficulty sleeping, research additional strategies to help you get the best sleep possible.

Be in nature

Being in nature and even seeing nature (including trees and green space) help to reduce stress and improve health.

The pack is on my back … I breathe the fresh air … walk the first steps of the trail and already life is better.

I sit by the ocean, the waves lapping at the shore … I sense … I am energized.

Laugh

One of my favourite songs is from the movie *Mary Poppins*: "I love to laugh, long and loud and clear, I love to laugh … it's getting worse every year!" What a fabulous song! I do love to laugh! The relatively new field of "laughter yoga" helps people obtain the benefits of laughter through laughter exercises. What might start as fake laughter soon becomes real laughter. Years ago I read that "laughter is internal jogging," and I am sure that this is one form of exercise that I can get hooked on!

Develop an attitude of gratitude

Feeling and expressing gratitude not only feels good, but can also benefit your body and your social network. Thank-you notes, flowers, sticky notes with positive comments … all help create a positive environment.

Keep a daily gratitude journal. At the end of each day, write three things that you are grateful for. Make it your goal to find something to be grateful for at work each day.

Enjoy "grateful" music. One of my other favourite songs is "What a Wonderful World." I joke that when my husband, Ted, and I die, one of our tombstones will read "What a wonderful world" and the other one, to the right, will read "But the best is yet to come!"

Create a transition ritual between work and home

Create a ritual that is a clear divider between work and home. Play a certain type of music when you are going home, change clothes once you arrive home, or routinely go for a walk after work. The important part is sending your mind a clear message that "work is over, leave the concerns behind." Regular use of this type of ritual will help you shift from a work mindset to a home mindset. If your home is busy and full, try to create a few minutes of peace before entering the door.

I placed a bird feeder in my backyard. When I get home I sit and relax for 5 to 10 minutes by the feeder before seeing the family.

I listen to relaxing music on the way home to transition gently into the next phase of my day.

Practise mindfulness

Mindfulness is one of the most effective strategies for reducing compassion fatigue. This stress reduction approach, developed over 30 years ago by Jon Kabat Zinn, a professor of medicine, is based on the practice of being present in the moment. That may sound simple, yet it can be surprisingly difficult to achieve at first! Here are some directions for achieving mindfulness.

An exercise in mindfulness

> Pick a quiet space where you will not be disturbed for the next 5 to 10 minutes. Sit comfortably, or lie down on the floor.
>
> Close your eyes, and focus on the feeling of the air coming in and out of your nostrils. There is no need to breathe in a special way, just notice what you notice.
>
> Unless you are very tired (in which case you will probably fall asleep), you might find yourself distracted by a million thoughts. Don't worry—that's normal. Just gently bring your mind back to noticing the air coming in and out of your nostrils.
>
> You may need to bring yourself back to the present a thousand times during the 10 minutes. That's all right; simply bring yourself back as often as you need. If you do this regularly, over time being mindful becomes second nature and can bring you to a state of calm and relaxation in a matter of seconds.

You can apply this practice to your daily tasks and do them in a mindful way. For example, when you are washing dishes, instead of having the television or radio on, pay attention to the warm water on your hands, the soap bubbles, the pot you are scrubbing.

Consider using coaching or counselling resources

As a society, we bring who we are and what we know to work, and then we use the experiences that happen at work to further our learning. Coaching, counselling, and feedback from supervisors can help you learn from your work experiences. You may have your own counselling support, or you may want to obtain support through the Employee Assistance Program. If you have not accessed counselling through the program, consider doing so. Many companies provide this service to employees, yet often the resource is not used.

Coaching is an emerging field. Coaches use a positive, strengths-based approach to help their clients achieve personal and professional growth. I was first introduced to coaching when a friend needed a guinea pig for part of her coaching training program. I was thrilled to assist. You may be able to access coaches through a coaching school; you could offer to help the coaching students learn. Coaching is frequently provided by telephone, so you do not need to live in the same geographic area as the coach. Distance coaching can be especially useful for PSWs who live in isolated communities.

Shake it up

As you reflect on and review your life and your work, you may feel a need for a change. It may be as simple as asking for a new assignment or a transfer to a new unit, or you may need to work for a different company or employer. You may want to decrease the number of hours you work in a week or the number of hours you work as a caregiver in a week. Maybe you just want to take a few months off from caregiving. You may be energized by doing totally different work, for example, in a flower shop or a grocery store.

Closing Thoughts

Self-care is essential to maintaining your health when working with the dying. Compassion fatigue can be a normal consequence of working with people experiencing life-threatening diseases. The key strategy is to notice where you are in terms of compassion fatigue and get help and support before you are suffering from total emotional exhaustion.

Care for yourself as well as you care for others. Access social and counselling support, enjoy opportunities for further education, and refuel regularly. When you are fatigued, step back, reflect, shake things up a bit, and get some extra support. Let your work as a caregiver strengthen you and enrich your life.

In closing, I share a favourite poem by Deanna Edwards, a singer and songwriter who made it her profession to help other people through music.

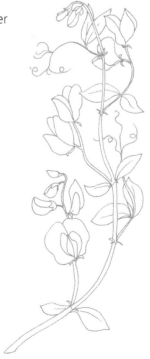

Teach Me to Die

Teach me to die,
Hold on to my hand
I have so many questions,
Things I don't understand

Teach me to die
Give all you can give
If you teach me of dying
I'll teach you to live

Appendix A:
Medications for Managing Symptoms[1]

Medications used to relieve pain are divided into three categories, based on their function: non-opioid analgesics, adjuvant analgesics, and opioid analgesics.

Non-Opioid Analgesics

Analgesics relieve pain through the peripheral nervous system. Acetaminophen is an example of a commonly used analgesic. Mild pain can often be treated using regular doses of acetaminophen.

Anti-inflammatory medications (e.g., ibuprofen) decrease local tissue inflammation, which in turn decreases the frequency and size of pain signals.

Sometimes people get better pain relief when they receive alternating doses of acetaminophen and ibuprofen.

If pain increases, it may be helpful to add in an adjuvant analgesic or an opioid.

Adjuvant Analgesics

The word "adjuvant" means "helpful" or "a helpful person or thing." Adjuvants are medications that, although used to treat other symptoms, relieve pain as a secondary function. Below are some examples of adjuvant medications:

Steroid medications (e.g., prednisone, dexamethasone) decrease inflammation and swelling around a tumour. This relieves pressure on tissues and consequently decreases pain. Steroids can prevent or decrease post-radiation pain caused by swelling in the radiated area.

Anticonvulsant medications (e.g., gabapentin) work by decreasing the excitability of nerves and thereby decreasing the number of pain signals sent to the brain. They are often used to decrease neuropathic (nerve) pain.

Antispasmodics (e.g., hyoscine butylbromide) relieve pain by decreasing muscle spasms. These medications are useful for bladder spasms or intestinal spasms.

---

1 The information in this appendix is provided so that you will be more aware and comfortable when medications are used to manage symptoms. Your scope of practice will determine whether or not your employer will require you to know this information.

Antidepressant medications (e.g., amitriptyline) can be effective at decreasing neuropathic pain if used at low doses.

Antibiotics (e.g., nitrofurantoin) can reduce pain by treating infections. For example, treating a bladder infection with an antibiotic can decrease pain felt when voiding.

Opioid Analgesics

Opioids[2] are crucial for relieving severe pain, which they do by decreasing the number and size of pain signals reaching the brain. The amount of opioid administered is increased or decreased to find the dose that is effective for the person. These drugs are administered regularly to provide steady pain control. The sections below discuss appropriate ways to use opioids for managing pain, the fears and concerns dying people and their families express about using opioids, and the side effects of opioids.

Principles for Using Opioids to Manage Pain

The opioid level in the blood must be greater than the person's pain relief threshold. Each person has a pain relief threshold that medications must surpass before their pain is relieved. The pain relief threshold is different in each person and changes over time and with different activities.

The opioid dose must be titrated to meet the needs of the person. The most effective dose of opioid is the dose that surpasses the person's pain relief threshold. Because this threshold is different for each person, the opioid is titrated (increased or decreased in a step-wise manner) to determine the correct dose of opioid for the particular person at a given time. This process of titrating opioids will result in the most effective dose of opioids with the fewest side effects.

Regular doses of opioids are needed to maintain pain relief. Regular doses maintain steady levels of opioids in the bloodstream, with the result that pain is controlled and the person remains comfortable. Opioids must be given regularly—every 4 hours for short-acting opioids, every 12 hours for most long-acting opioids, and every 72 hours for transdermal fentanyl patches. Preventing pain from returning and escalating is more effective and efficient than waiting until the person is in pain again before giving another opioid dose. Therefore, a person might have to be woken up at night and administered medication.

Breakthrough doses are administered when regular doses fail to control pain. When regular doses of opioids do not control pain, an extra dose (breakthrough dose) is given to manage pain. Breakthrough doses are used when pain increases,

---

2 Currently, health care professionals refer to these medications as "opioids" rather than "narcotics." The term "narcotics" is commonly used to refer to illegal street drugs and also to drugs that induce sleep, and therefore the term is inappropriate in the context of HPC.

before a painful procedure or stressful event, after a painful incident, and when titrating the correct regular dose. Breakthrough doses are also known as incident doses, rescue doses, booster doses, and bolus or interim doses.

The route of opioid administration should be changed when necessary. As a person's health declines, they may not be able to take medications by mouth, for example, if they have difficulty swallowing. Report swallowing problems to the nurse and work with the family and care facility to prepare for and choose a different route of administration.

Fears and Misconceptions about Opioids

Dying people, their family, and staff may express fears and misconceptions about using opioids for managing pain in the dying person. The most common fears and misconceptions about using opioids are discussed below.

Symbolism. *If he is taking morphine, it means he is dying.*

Some people believe that when a person is given morphine (or another opioid), death must be imminent. This misperception may have developed when only people who were about to die were given opioids.

Currently, many people receive opioids early in the disease process to manage their pain. Doses are increased or decreased to control symptoms and side effects. Current studies suggest that patients who receive good palliative care (which includes pain control) live longer than those who do not.

Tolerance. *If he becomes used to this dose of medication, then it will not work for him when his pain increases.*

Tolerance occurs when the body requires more of the same medication to reach the person's pain relief threshold. Tolerance develops in people at different rates. Therefore, if a person develops tolerance to the current dose of opioids, the dose will need to be increased. There is no limit to the amount of opioid that can be used to treat pain caused by cancer.

Dependence. *He will become dependent on these medications.*

Physical dependence occurs when the body becomes accustomed to taking a specific amount of medication. If the person's pain is relieved (e.g., with surgery), the medication can be withdrawn slowly by a weaning process to prevent withdrawal symptoms. This is *not* considered addiction.

Addiction. *I don't want to become addicted.*

Addiction is rarely an issue for people who are receiving opioids under a doctor's supervision to treat pain caused by a life-threatening illness, and who do not have a prior history of addiction. Addiction is a psychological issue. Addiction involves the intentional use of drugs for effects other than pain management. A person who is addicted usually has both an overwhelming preoccupation to take more medication than is required to manage the pain and displays compulsive drug-seeking behaviours.

When a person is in pain, the body uses opioids and responds differently to them than when the person is not in pain. Practically speaking, addiction caused by long-term opioid use in palliative care is rare.

Respiratory depression. *It might slow her breathing down, and then she won't get enough oxygen.*

Pain is a powerful respiratory stimulant. This explains why opioids are ineffective at decreasing respiration rates when a person is in pain. Only when opioid doses exceed the amount of medication needed to control pain will the opioid cause respiration to start to slow. If respiratory depression is suspected, the health care team has sufficient time to re-evaluate the opioid dose. As the person's body adjusts to the opioid, this side effect usually subsides. There is usually a significant difference between the therapeutic dose to control pain and a dose sufficient to stop respiration. If a patient's breathing does slow significantly, caregivers may need to consider whether the period of apnea (not breathing) might be a sign that the individual could be dying imminently. As with other concerns, caregivers can and should discuss their concerns about possible respiratory depression with the health care team.

When a dying person or their family members talk about their concerns regarding opioids, you can connect them with appropriate members of the health care team who can provide information about the use of medication and support informed decision making and goal setting

Common Side Effects of Opioids

People may experience side effects when taking opioids. Common side effects include constipation, nausea and vomiting, confusion or delirium, and drowsiness. Occasionally opioid toxicity may occur. Less common side effects include a dry, sore mouth, itchiness, urinary retention or hesitancy, sweating, and myoclonus (muscle twitching or jerking). One way to minimize the side effects is to encourage fluid intake if the person is able to swallow.

Constipation. Opioids decrease motility in the intestines and cause constipation. Most people develop constipation when taking opioids. Therefore, the doctor should prescribe laxatives when starting a person on opioids.

Nausea and vomiting. These symptoms can occur when a person initially begins taking opioids or after several days or weeks of taking opioids. If the nausea or vomiting starts soon after the opioid is administered, this side effect may be triggered by the brain recognizing the opioid in the bloodstream and trying to get rid of it. If the side effect occurs several days after starting the opioid, beginning with decreased appetite at lunchtime and then the vomiting of undigested food at dinnertime, the opioid may be causing the digestive process to slow down, resulting in poor digestion and the vomiting of undigested food. Decreased motility in the intestines may be causing constipation, which may in turn cause nausea and vomiting.

Opioid doses need to be adjusted depending on what is occurring in the person's body. The information the PSW gathers will help the health care team assess what medication will best meet the needs of the person.

Confusion or delirium. Confusion or delirium, illusions, and increased dreaming can result from the use of opioids. Some people are more susceptible than others to these side effects. If opioids are contributing to confusion or delirium, a lower dose of opioids or less frequent increases in the dose may help. For some people, switching to a different opioid helps. Some people may need other medications (e.g., haloperidol) to reduce or control the confusion or delirium, especially if they are restless or agitated. More information is available in the section on delirium in Chapter 4.

Drowsiness. When a person initially takes an opioid or the dose is increased, they can expect to be drowsy for the first few days. It is helpful to inform both the person and their family about possible drowsiness so that they are not surprised by it. Reassure them that drowsiness when starting opioids is normal and the drowsiness will decrease after a few days. Perhaps it occurs because the person is more comfortable now that the pain is controlled, so the person is able catch up on previously missed sleep. Sleeping provides time for the body to adjust to the new medication.

The health care team may also explain to the patient and family that when opioids are started early in the disease process, the person has the opportunity to respond to the medication and overcome the side effects. However, if the medication is started late in the disease process, closer to death, then the person will be sleeping more as a result of the dying process, so drowsiness might not decrease in the coming days. This lack of responsiveness will not be due to the opioid.

As part of their care for the dying person, PSWs should watch for side effects of opioid use and record and report them if and when they occur. Comfort measures relating to these symptoms are discussed in Chapter 4.

Opioid toxicity. Occasionally a person who is taking opioids develops opioid toxicity: the by-products of the opioids build up in the person's bloodstream. This usually occurs when a person takes high doses of opioids over a long time, or if the kidneys are not able to excrete the medication. Symptoms of opioid toxicity are different from the normal side effects and include delirium, myoclonus, and hyperalgesia—hypersensitivity to pain—such as sensitivity to even gentle touches. PSWs should record and report any of these symptoms, but the physician and nurse will decide what their cause is.

Any sudden or sharp increase in drowsiness or other symptoms could indicate a change in the person's general condition and the need for reassessment by the physician or nurse.

Appendix B:
Supporting Children Whose Loved One Is Dying

Many people find it challenging to support a child when a person close to them is dying or has died. In North America, death and dying have moved out of the home and into hospitals and long-term care facilities. This separation of dying and death from ordinary life has raised more issues than it has solved. When the dying process happens behind closed doors, adults may separate children from their dying loved one, often with the unintended effect of interfering with children's ability to say goodbye to the person. In addition, the separation denies children the opportunity to learn about death, one of life's greatest teachers. Current research-based principles on supporting children whose loved one is dying suggest that they should be included and communication with them should be open and honest.

Applying the principles discussed below can help health care providers and families feel more confident when supporting children whose loved one is dying, as well as help children in their grieving process.

Principles for Supporting Children Whose Loved One Is Dying

Including Children

People often ask questions such as "Should my daughter visit her grandfather who is dying?" Children benefit by having the choice to visit dying friends and family members. Children of all ages should be asked whether they want to visit and should be allowed to participate to the extent that they are comfortable doing so.

Preparing Children

Some parents are hesitant to let a child visit a dying person due to concerns that the person's appearance or the equipment in the person's room may frighten the child. Preparing a child to visit their loved one will help make the experience a positive one. Before the visit, talk with the child about the following:
- How the person's room will look
- The equipment in the room, the lights on the equipment, and the sounds it makes

- How their loved one looks now, including describing any dramatic changes, such as weight loss, hair loss, or pallor, since the child last saw the person (a child could be shocked by seeing a person who customarily wears dentures without them)
- The rules for visitors
- What the child is allowed to do in the presence of, say to, or talk about with the dying person
- What will happen during the visit (e.g., both laughter and tears may occur)

Being Honest

Adults may try to protect children from the news that a family member is dying. However, most children sense when something is wrong in the family, and if they are not told the truth, they invent a story to explain what is wrong. Quite often their imaginations create scenarios that are worse than reality. This means that withholding the news that a family member is dying tends to be more frightening than the truth, and denies children access to accurate information and appropriate emotional support. When children sense they have not been told the truth or they learn the truth after the fact, their sense of security and ability to trust the adults around them are damaged.

Inviting Participation in Caregiving

Children may want to participate in caregiving but probably will not know what to do or how to help. A child can be included in caregiving by inviting them to
- Help with personal care, such as mouth care and applying nail polish or skin moisturizer
- Help create a comfortable atmosphere by means of music, decorations, storytelling, or reminiscing
- Share daily events, do homework, or do other quiet activities at the bedside
- Sit quietly at the bedside and hold hands with their loved one

Inviting Questions

Children often have many questions about what is happening to their dying family member and the care that the person is receiving. It is important to invite children to ask questions with statements such as "You are welcome to ask me any questions."

When a child asks questions, be prepared to repeat your answers, as the child may ask the same questions repeatedly. If you do not have an answer, be honest and tell the child that you do not know the answer. If someone else on the care team or in the family might know the answer to the question, ask that person to help the child.

Whatever questions children ask, thank them for asking and let them know that their questions are good ones. Also encourage children to share their questions about dying and death with other caregivers.

Using Correct Language

In an effort to protect children, adults often avoid using the name of the disease by instead saying that the person is sick or has an illness. This can confuse children. When an adult says, "Your grandma is sick and will die," the child may start to think that anyone who is sick will die. Using correct language that names the illness (e.g., "Your grandma has leukemia") will help prevent such confusion.

It is also common for adults to avoid using certain words around children, specifically "dying," "death," and "died," and substitute other words, such as "passing" or "passed away." Substituting words can confuse children. Use the correct language and avoid using unclear terms such as those below to describe dying and death:

- "Passing" or "passed away." These terms do not indicate what has happened to the person and will be difficult for children to understand.
- "Mommy went to a better place." Children may interpret this to mean that Mommy chose to leave the family and go somewhere else.
- "We lost Grandpa." Children frequently lose things and find them later. Saying that someone is lost may lead children to believe the person will be found later.
- "Dad will never get better." This phrase doesn't accurately indicate that Dad is dying. Children may think that Dad will live forever in his current state of functioning.
- "It's like a big sleep." This phrase may make children believe that falling asleep is dying and therefore cause them to fear falling asleep.

The best way to proceed is to use the correct language, such as "death", "dying" and "died," rather than vague phrases that children may misinterpret. This will help children develop an understanding of death. Death can be explained as "When a body stops working and will never work again."

Understanding Children's Concerns: The Three C's

Children who whose loved one is dying often have three concerns, referred to here as "the three C's":

1. Did I cause it?
Children often feel more responsible for what is happening around them than adults realize. If, for example, the child had been angry with the person who is dying, the child may believe they caused the dying to happen or that it is a punishment for their misbehaviour. Even if a child shows no signs of feeling responsible for the illness, it is important to let the child know that nothing they did or thought caused or can cause illness or death.

2. Can I catch it?
Children often think that all illnesses are like the common cold, the flu, or chicken pox and can be spread from one person to another. It helps to explain to children that diseases that are not contagious, such as amyotrophic lateral sclerosis and can-

cer, or dying of old age, do not work this way—one person cannot catch them from another person.

3. Who will take care of me?
If child's parent or guardian is dying, it is important that the parents or guardians let the child know who will take care of them following the person's death.

Recognizing Children's Grief

Children, like adults, have a range of responses to death and dying. Adults are often surprised to see children who are very upset one moment about a family member's dying, and then playing happily the next. It is important to allow children, like all people, to express their sorrow in their own way and in their own time. Children will naturally regulate the amount of time they spend experiencing intense emotions by taking breaks from the feelings through play and continuing to enjoy life. It is also important to realize that because children get up from crying and go out to play, they are not over their grief but rather are dealing with it bit by bit, as they are able.

Children's grief may include the following:
- Sleep disturbances
- Stomach aches and headaches
- Difficulty concentrating in school
- Angry outbursts
- Fears about seemingly unrelated things

Grieving Together

Adults who hide their emotions from children in an effort to protect them may inadvertently teach them that grief should be hidden.

It is important for kids to know that all of the feelings they are experiencing are normal, and that adults experience them too.

Grief can be described to children as "all of the feelings people experience when someone is dying or has died. This includes being sad, mad, worried, and lonely, as well as being happy and continuing to enjoy life."

Children learn how to grieve by watching the adults around them. PSWs can let families know that it is okay for them to cry together, be mad together, and be sad together, and that moments of happiness and laughter are all part of the process. Sometimes children will ask questions or make comments that are surprising or disturbing to other people. It is important that children are supported regardless of whether what they say is politically correct.

Supporting children through the death of someone they care about can be a heart-breaking experience during what is already a difficult time. However, death is an inevitable part of life and ultimately not something from which children can be protected. Adults can help prepare children for a loved one's death by including children at the bedside and providing them with ongoing emotional support. Preparing kids for dying and death can help prepare them for life and living. By doing this, health care professionals, parents and guardians, and other family members can play a powerful role in shaping children's experience of the death while at the same time equipping them to deal with future adversity.

Appendix C:
Palliative Performance Scale

PPS Level	Ambulation	Activity & Evidence of Disease	Self-Care	Intake	Conscious Level
		Palliative Performance Scale (PPSv2) version 2			
100%	Full	Normal activity & work No evidence of disease	Full	Normal	Full
90%	Full	Normal activity & work Some evidence of disease	Full	Normal	Full
80%	Full	Normal activity with effort Some evidence of disease	Full	Normal or reduced	Full
70%	Reduced	Unable normal job/work Significant disease	Full	Normal or reduced	Full
60%	Reduced	Unable hobby/house work Significant disease	Occasional assistance necessary	Normal or reduced	Full or Confusion
50%	Mainly Sit/Lie	Unable to do any work Extensive disease	Considerable assistance required	Normal or reduced	Full or Confusion
40%	Mainly in Bed	Unable to do most activity Extensive disease	Mainly assistance	Normal or reduced	Full or Drowsy +/– Confusion
30%	Totally Bed Bound	Unable to do any activity Extensive disease	Total Care	Normal or reduced	Full or Drowsy +/– Confusion
20%	Totally Bed Bound	Unable to do any activity Extensive disease	Total Care	Minimal to sips	Full or Drowsy +/– Confusion
10%	Totally Bed Bound	Unable to do any activity Extensive disease	Total Care	Mouth care only	Drowsy or Coma +/– Confusion
0%	Death	—	—	—	—

Reproduced with permission. Copyright Victoria Hospice Society, BC, Canada (2001) www.victoriahospice.org.

Instructions for Use of PPS
(see also definition of terms)

1. PPS scores are determined by reading horizontally at each level to find a 'best fit' for the patient which is then assigned as the PPS% score.

2. Begin at the left column and read downwards until the appropriate ambulation level is reached, then read across to the next column and downwards again until the activity/evidence of disease is located. These steps are repeated until all five columns are covered before assigning the actual PPS for that patient. In this way, 'leftward' columns (columns to the left of any specific column) are 'stronger' determinants and generally take precedence over others.

   Example 1: A patient who spends the majority of the day sitting or lying down due to fatigue from advanced disease and requires considerable assistance to walk even for short distances but who is otherwise fully conscious level with good intake would be scored at PPS 50%.

Example 2: A patient who has become paralyzed and quadriplegic requiring total care would be PPS 30%. Although this patient may be placed in a wheelchair (and perhaps seem initially to be at 50%), the score is 30% because he or she would be otherwise totally bed bound due to the disease or complication if it were not for caregivers providing total care including lift/transfer. The patient may have normal intake and full conscious level.

Example 3: However, if the patient in example 2 was paraplegic and bed bound but still able to do some self-care such as feed themselves, then the PPS would be higher at 40 or 50% since he or she is not 'total care.'

3. PPS scores are in 10% increments only. Sometimes, there are several columns easily placed at one level but one or two which seem better at a higher or lower level. One then needs to make a 'best fit' decision. Choosing a 'half-fit' value of PPS 45%, for example, is not correct. The combination of clinical judgment and 'leftward precedence' is used to determine whether 40% or 50% is the more accurate score for that patient.

4. PPS may be used for several purposes. First, it is an excellent communication tool for quickly describing a patient's current functional level. Second, it may have value in criteria for workload assessment or other measurements and comparisons. Finally, it appears to have prognostic value.

Definition of Terms for PPS

As noted below, some of the terms have similar meanings with the differences being more readily apparent as one reads horizontally across each row to find an overall 'best fit' using all five columns.

1. Ambulation

The items '**mainly sit/lie**,' '**mainly in bed**,' and '**totally bed bound**' are clearly similar. The subtle differences are related to items in the self-care column. For example, 'totally bed 'bound' at PPS 30% is due to either profound weakness or paralysis such that the patient not only can't get out of bed but is also unable to do any self-care. The difference between 'sit/lie' and 'bed' is proportionate to the amount of time the patient is able to sit up vs need to lie down.

'Reduced ambulation' is located at the PPS 70% and PPS 60% level. By using the adjacent column, the reduction of ambulation is tied to inability to carry out their normal job, work occupation or some hobbies or housework activities. The person is still able to walk and transfer on their own but at PPS 60% needs occasional assistance.

2. Activity & Extent of disease

'**Some**,' '**significant**,' and '**extensive**' disease refer to physical and investigative evidence which shows degrees of progression. For example in breast cancer, a local recurrence would imply 'some' disease, one or two metastases in the lung or bone would imply 'significant' disease, whereas multiple metastases in lung, bone, liver, brain, hypercalcemia or other major complications would be 'extensive' disease. The extent may also refer to progression of disease despite active treatments. Using PPS in AIDS, 'some' may mean the shift from HIV to AIDS, 'significant' implies progression in physical decline, new or difficult symptoms and laboratory findings with low counts. 'Extensive' refers to one or more serious complications with or without continuation of active antiretrovirals, antibiotics, etc.

The above extent of disease is also judged in context with the ability to maintain one's work and hobbies or activities. Decline in activity may mean the person still plays golf but reduces from playing 18 holes to 9 holes, or just a par 3, or to backyard putting. People who enjoy walking will gradually reduce the distance covered, although they may continue trying, sometimes even close to death (e.g. trying to walk the halls).

3. Self-Care

'**Occasional assistance**' means that most of the time patients are able to transfer out of bed, walk, wash, toilet and eat by their own means, but that on occasion (perhaps once daily or a few times weekly) they require minor assistance.

'**Considerable assistance**' means that regularly every day the patient needs help, usually by one person, to do some of the activities noted above. For example, the person needs help to get to the bathroom but is then able to brush his or her teeth or wash at least hands and face. Food will often need to be cut into edible sizes but the patient is then able to eat of his or her own accord.

'**Mainly assistance**' is a further extension of 'considerable.' Using the above example, the patient now needs help getting up but also needs assistance washing his face and shaving, but can usually eat with minimal or no help. This may fluctuate according to fatigue during the day.

'**Total care**' means that the patient is completely unable to eat without help, toilet or do any self-care. Depending on the clinical situation, the patient may or may not be able to chew and swallow food once prepared and fed to him or her.

4. Intake

Changes in intake are quite obvious with '**normal intake**' referring to the person's usual eating habits while healthy. '**Reduced**' means any reduction from that and is highly variable according to the unique individual circumstances. '**Minimal**' refers to very small amounts, usually pureed or liquid, which are well below nutritional sustenance.

5. Conscious Level

'**Full consciousness**' implies full alertness and orientation with good cognitive abilities in various domains of thinking, memory, etc. '**Confusion**' is used to denote presence of either delirium or dementia and is a reduced level of consciousness. It may be mild, moderate or severe with multiple possible etiologies. '**Drowsiness**' implies either fatigue, drug side effects, delirium or closeness to death and is sometimes included in the term stupor. '**Coma**' in this context is the absence of response to verbal or physical stimuli; some reflexes may or may not remain. The depth of coma may fluctuate throughout a 24 hour period.

The Palliative Performance Scale version 2 (PPSv2) tool is copyright to Victoria Hospice Society and replaces the first PPS published in 1996 [J Pall Care 9(4): 26-32]. It cannot be altered or used in any way other than as intended and described here. Programs may use PPSv2 with appropriate recognition. Available in electronic Word format by email request to edu.hospice@viha.ca. Correspondence should be sent to Medical Director, Victoria Hospice Society, 1952 Bay Street, Victoria, BC, V8R 1J8, Canada

Palliative Performance Scale (PPSv2) version 2. Medical Care of the Dying, 4th ed.; p. 121.
©Victoria Hospice Society, 2006.

Appendix D:
Resources

References

Albom, M. *Tuesdays with Morrie: An Old Man, a Young Man, and Life's Greatest Lesson.* New York: Random House, 1997.

Bern-Klug, M. "The Ambiguous Dying Syndrome." *Health and Social Work* 29, no. 1 (2004): 55–65.

Bruera, E., et al. "Parenteral Hydration in Patients with Advanced Cancer: A Multicenter, Double-Blind, Placebo-Controlled Randomized Trial." *Journal of Clinical Oncology* 31, no. 1 (2013): 111–118.

Buckman, R. *I Don't Know What to Say: How to Help and Support Someone Who Is Dying.* Toronto. Key Porter Books, 2005.

Cairns, M., M. Thomson, and W. Wainwright. *Transitions in Dying and Bereavement: A Psychosocial Guide for Hospice and Palliative Care.* Baltimore, MD: Health Professions Press, 2003.

Callanan, M., and P. Kelley. *Final Gifts: Understanding the Special Awareness, Needs, and Communications of the Dying.* Toronto: Bantam Books, 1993.

Canadian Hospice Palliative Care Association. *A Model to Guide Hospice Palliative Care: Based on National Principles and Norms of Practice,* revised and condensed ed., 2013. http://www.chpca.net/media/319547/norms-of-practice-eng-web.pdf.

Canadian Hospice Palliative Care Association. Fact Sheet—Hospice Palliative Care in Canada. http://www.chpca.net/media/330558/Fact_Sheet_HPC_in_Canada%20 Spring%202014%20Final.pdf.

Canadian Virtual Hospice. http://virtualhospice.org/.

Colleges and Institutes Canada. Canadian Educational Standards for Personal Care Providers, 2012. http://www.collegesinstitutes.ca/what-we-do/canadian-partnerships/ national-educational-standards-for-personal-care-providers/.

Dignity in Care. The Patient Dignity Question. http://dignityincare.ca/en/toolkit. html#The_Patient_Dignity_Question.

Downing, M., and W. Wainwright. *Medical Care of the Dying*, 4th ed. Victoria, BC: Victoria Hospice, 2006.

Fraser Health. Fraser Health Symptom Assessment Acronym, Symptom Guidelines. 2006. http://www.fraserhealth.ca/media/SymptomAssessmentRevised_Sept09.pdf.

Initiative for a Palliative Approach in Nursing (iPANEL). *Evidence and Leadership.* BC: University of Victoria. http://www.ipanel.ca/.

LaGrand, L. *Gifts from the Unknown: Using Extraordinary Experiences to Cope with Loss and Change.* San Jose: Author's Choice Press, 2001.

Martin, T., and K. Doka. *Men Don't Cry, Women Do: Transcending Gender Stereotypes of Grief.* New York: Brunner Mazel/Taylor and Francis, 2000.

Nouwen, H. *The Way of the Heart: Desert Spirituality and Contemporary Ministry.* New York: Seabury Press, 1981, 34.

Ontario Ministry of Training, Colleges and Universities. *Personal Support Worker Program Standard.* 2014. http://www.tcu.gov.on.ca/pepg/audiences/colleges/progstan/health/41469.pdf.

O'Rourke, M., and E. Dufour. *Embracing the End of Life: Help for Those Who Accompany the Dying.* Toronto: Novalis, 2012.

Palliative Alliance (Quality Palliative Care in Long Term Care). http://www.palliativealliance.ca/.

Remen, R.N. *Kitchen Table Wisdom: Stories That Heal.* New York: Putnam, 1997.

Schwalbe, W. *The End of Your Life Book Club.* New York: First Vintage Books, 2012.

Speak Up: Advance Care Planning in Canada. http://www.advancecareplanning.ca/.

Soelle, D. *Suffering.* Philadelphia: Fortress Press, 1975, 76.

Temel, J.S., et al. "Early Palliative Care for Patients with Metastatic Non-Small-Cell Lung Cancer." *New England Journal of Medicine* 363, no. 8 (2010): 733–742.

Victoria Hospice. Palliative Performance Scale. http://www.victoriahospice.org/sites/default/files/pps_english.pdf.

Warden, V., A.C. Hurley, and L. Volicer. "Development and Psychometric Evaluation of the Pain Assessment in Advanced Dementia (PAINAD) Scale." *Journal of the American Medical Directors Association* 4, no. 1 (2003): 9–15.

Williams, M. *The* Velveteen *Rabbit.* http://digital.library.upenn.edu/women/williams/rabbit/rabbit.html.

Recommended Reading for Personal Support Workers

Books

Buckman, R. *I Don't Know What to Say: How to Help and Support Someone Who Is Dying*. Toronto: Key Porter Books, 2005.

Callanan, M., and P. Kelley. *Final Gifts: Understanding the Special Awareness, Needs, and Communications of the Dying*. Toronto: Bantam Books, 1993.

Joseph, E. *In the Slender Margin: The Intimate Strangeness of Dying*. Toronto: Harper-Collins, 2014. (This book is a journey into the land of death and dying seen through the lens of art and the imagination.)

Remen, R.N. *Kitchen Table Wisdom: Stories That Heal*. New York: Putnam, 1997.

Websites

Canadian Hospice Palliative Care Association. http://www.chpca.net/

Canadian Virtual Hospice. http://virtualhospice.ca

Life and Death Matters. http://www.lifeanddeathmatters.ca/

Speak Up: Advance Care Planning in Canada. http://www.advancecareplanning.ca/

The Way Forward: An Integrated Palliative Approach to Care. http://www.hpcintegration.ca/

Your provincial hospice palliative care association

Index

integrating, 28

palliative care
defined for this book, 30
origins, 25
unit, 30

palliative consult team, 30

Palliative Performance Scale (PPS), 50–51. *See also* **Tools, PPS**

Parkinson's Disease
pattern of dying, 18, 20

patterns
of dying, 14
slow decline, 20
steady decline, 16
stuttering decline, 18
sudden death, 15

Personal Support Worker
role on the Health Care Team, 34
ways to provide support, 36

positioning
to manage difficult breathing, 88
to manage nausea/vomiting, 98
to manage pain, 110
with congested breathing, 169
with unresponsiveness, 167

process
of dying, 23

psychosocial support, 126–149
dementia, 124
certainties, 125
interventions, 125
signs that death is near, 125
uncertainties, 124
family, 128
hope, 127
independence, 126
information sharing, 122–125
transitions with dying, 119

Q

quality of life
with HPC, 25

questions
asked by family during last days and hours, 155
sample responses, 153
how to answer during last days and hours, 153
questions family ask, 153
that family ask about support, 155
to address family's understanding, 154
to ask about rituals, 157

Questions. *See* **Sample Questions**

R

reassurance
after delirium, 83
during delirium, 82
false, 38

recording and reporting, 54
sample record, 55
sample report, 55
samples, 57

reflection
activities for self-care, 6

refuelling
care-giver, 199

residential hospice, 30

respect
cultural and spiritual, 4

respiration
signs of difficult breathing. *See* breathing; difficult

rituals
door openers to conversations about, 157

roadblocks to communicating
Fix-It Trap, 39
judging, labelling, 39
offering sympathy, 38
platitudes, 38
praising, 38
to communication, 37

roller coaster
pattern of decline, 18

S

Sample Questions, 52–53. *See also* **Tools; List of Samples Questions**
and pain, 104
reference, 49

Saunders, Cicely, 25

self-awareness, 4
definition, 4

self-care, 196–203
and learning, 199
and self-awareness, 196
and social network, 198
boundaries and, 8
importance when caring for the dying, 191
maintaining boundaries, 197
PPS indicator, 50
refuelling, 199

self-reflection
understanding your baggage, 2

sharing information
uncertainty with transitions, 122

side effects
opioids, 61–62

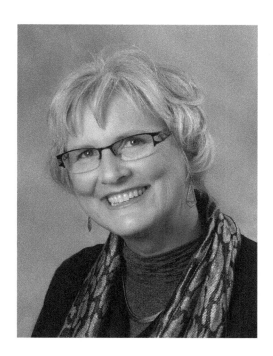

About the Author

Kath is a hospice palliative care nurse, a thanatologist (which means that she specializes in death, dying, and bereavement), an educator, a mom, and a nana.

She has a love for education that is engaging, delicious, and digestible. Her passion is to develop and provide excellent resources (based on current research and best practice) to help front line caregivers provide excellent care for the dying and their family.

Kath appreciates hearing about your experiences and receiving feedback. You can email Kath from the Life and Death Matters website, www.lifeanddeathmatters.ca.

CPSIA information can be obtained
at www.ICGtesting.com
Printed in the USA
LVHW070624240719
625063LV00022B/243/P